# Mediterr: Diet for Beginners

*Form new Mini Habits, Increase Longevity, and Burn fat Forever with the Best solution to a Paleo or Keto Diet! (complete Weight Loss Guide, Intermittent Fasting tips)*

**By**
**Serena Baker**

# Table of Contents

assurance regarding its prolonged validity or interim quality. Trademarks that are mentioned are done without written consent and can in no way be considered an endorsement from the trademark holder.

# Introduction

Congratulations on downloading *"Mediterranean Diet for Beginners,"* and thank you for doing so. By starting this book, you have shown an interest in changing your life for the better, and you should be applauded for this decision.

The following chapters will discuss everything you need to know to successfully begin incorporating the Mediterranean diet and lifestyle into your daily life. You'll find that there is so much more to this eating plan than food, though! The Mediterranean diet is a relaxed, low-stress, active, and social way of approaching life. By celebrating fresh, local, and whole foods, the people who inspired this diet have taught us that dieting does not have to make us feel like we are depriving ourselves of anything. You'll learn to feed yourself in a way that genuinely fuels your body from the inside out in a way that makes you feel alive and satisfied.

In this guide, you'll learn about the solid scientific research that went into the establishment of the Mediterranean diet, as the number one diet for long-term healthy living. You'll discover how to start approaching life as the Mediterranean people do, and how to begin shopping for food with a new perspective.
Finally, you'll also learn how to lose weight on the Mediterranean diet, and you'll get helpful hints for if you are having trouble losing weight. You'll even get a good breakdown of many of today's popular fad diets, from ketogenic to intermittent fasting. You'll learn how the Mediterranean diet stacks up against each one and how to compromise between this eating plan, and any others that are beneficial for you. This guide concludes with 20 mouth-watering and healthy Mediterranean recipes to get you started on your new way of life.

Every effort was made to ensure it is full of as much useful information as possible. So please, enjoy!

# Chapter 1: The Mediterranean Way of Life

An incredibly diverse group of countries encompasses the Mediterranean Sea. These countries include, but are not limited to the following: Italy, Morocco, France, Syria, Spain, Greece, and Egypt. Because there are so very many countries in this region, it is impossible to define a single "diet" that includes cuisines from the whole region. Instead, the Mediterranean diet contains the commonalities of these areas: namely, efforts to eat copious amounts of vegetables and fruits, whole grains, lentils, beans, fish and shellfish instead of meat, and plenty of olive oil. These components make up the heart of the Mediterranean eating plan.

**The Philosophy Behind the Mediterranean Diet**

The Mediterranean diet is not just another diet fad. Instead, it's a whole way of life – a way of life millions of people residing along the Mediterranean Sea have been thriving on for thousands of years. This lifestyle incorporates an array of flavorful and healthy ingredients, along with a different approach to life than the one to which most residents of the United States have become accustomed. There is so much more to the Mediterranean diet and lifestyle than just food. It's also about making small changes to your daily life that improve the overall quality of your health.

**Reducing Stress**

By and large, people living in Mediterranean countries tend to have less stress in their daily lives when compared to their American counterparts. They spend much more time enjoying meals with loved ones. They often relax and take a short nap after lunch. It's common to take a 2-hour break in the middle of the day to have lunch and take a nap. When scientists looked into this practice of a post-lunch rest, they realized that the people in this area have a good thing going. Recent research showed that regularly snoozing for a short time in the middle of the day reduced your risk of death from heart disease by 37 percent!

## The Effects of Stress

Doctors often neglect to counsel patients on the impact of chronic stress on long-term health during routine exams and office visits. This gap in information given to patients is unfortunate, since stress may be the most critical health risk factor faced by most of us! The issue with stress is that we cannot measure it in the same ways that we measure blood pressure or heart rate. It is a somewhat ambiguous and subjectively measured factor, especially since what causes stress for one person may not cause stress for another. Some people thrive on certain types of stress, like the pressure of looming deadlines and a fast-paced work environment. However, if one of those same people was to decide to start a family and have her first child, she might find herself overwhelmed by an entirely different type of stress. On the other hand, certain people seem like they are born to handle the everyday pressure of raising children, with all its unpredictability and sleepless nights; but if they suddenly entered a fast-paced work environment, they might lose their minds entirely.

No matter the source, chronic stress causes an increase in cortisol and adrenaline, which are stress hormones. These hormones are responsible for the rise in blood pressure. It also raises one's heart rate, making the formation of blood clots in the process. Research has proven that heart attacks are more likely to occur in individuals who face chronic stress. Moreover, certain people who are highly reactive and impatient are even more prone to cardiovascular problems.

## Daily Exercise

Besides lower stress levels in the Mediterranean culture, exercise is also part of everyday life. People do a lot of walking – and who wouldn't, with the beautiful weather and stunning views around the Mediterranean Sea? Whether it's waking up early to take a stroll, walking to the grocery store, gardening, or sweeping the yard, physical activity isn't given a second thought.

## Family Time

The family is a big part of the Mediterranean culture. Family get-togethers aren't just during the holidays or special events in this culture. They're held every few days or at least once a week, creating a special bond among everyone at the table.

# Chapter 2: The Mediterranean Diet in a Nutshell

In summary, the Mediterranean diet is a way of eating that combines whole non-processed foods and is rich in a wide variety of health-promoting vitamins and nutrients. Countless health and dietary experts recognize it as the ideal nutritional plan for long-term heart health and weight control – in fact, multiple clinical trials have demonstrated its benefits.

Many people who live along the Mediterranean coast don't think of their eating habits as a diet – it's just their way of life. Eating fresh, plant-based ingredients and getting regular physical activity is how they've lived for thousands of years.

There's no subscription to prepackaged Mediterranean diet meals you can buy, and there isn't a calorie meal plan you have to follow. You don't have to ban any food group, and you don't have to avoid carbs. Instead, you'll be more conscious and mindful of how you eat every day – just like the millions of people along the Mediterranean Sea.

## How the Mediterranean Diet Became Popular

This way of eating was first brought to light by American scientist Dr. Ancel Keys. In the late 1950s, Keys conducted the Seven Countries Study, which followed the diet and lifestyle habits of participants in seven different countries – the Netherlands, Finland, Japan, Yugoslavia (formerly), Italy, and the United States.

Keys' findings showed that eating habits, types of fat consumption, and physical activity greatly decreased the study participants' risk of cardiovascular disease. What's more, it highlighted the fact that the people who had already embraced this diet and lifestyle lived along the Mediterranean Sea. Since Keys' work, hundreds of other studies have been conducted and continue to support his findings of the many benefits of the Mediterranean diet. You'll read more about the research of Keys and other scientists in Chapter 3, "Who Should Consider the Mediterranean Diet and Why?

Not every single country along the Mediterranean eats the same way, but most do embrace many aspects of the Mediterranean diet as part of their culture and way of living. The type of food consumed differs based on country, culture, agriculture, and even regions within each country. This section of the book will give you an understanding of the essential parts of this diet.

Below the key components that combine to make this diet and lifestyle work:

- Eating fresh, in-season fruits and vegetables
- Reducing processed foods
- Using whole grains in everyday recipes
- Using "good" fats or unsaturated fats, from fish, extra virgin olive oil, nuts, and avocados.
- Eating moderate amounts of low-fat dairy such as Greek yogurt, which has lots of probiotics that are great for your digestive system, and cheese.
- Consuming lean protein from eggs, fish, poultry, and small amounts of red meat.
- Filling your diet with legumes, including beans, seeds, and nuts
- Using fresh and dried herbs and spices to boost flavor
- Drinking red wine, in moderation (This isn't necessary if you do not consume alcohol.)
- Getting daily exercise
- Reducing your stress level

- Making time for family

The above are some basic things to remember, but what's most important is to incorporate each item in a way that suits you, so you're more likely to continue to follow these tips.

# Creating a Mediterranean Table

Adapting your mindset to the Mediterranean diet certainly will be an adjustment if you are accustomed to how we typically approach food in the United States. In the Mediterranean diet, you'll encounter smaller portion sizes and get used to the idea of eating less meat overall defines a serving size. You'll also find that Mediterranean meals often include several dishes of equal importance, rather than the main dish with a few sides. The following recommendations can help guide you as you work to incorporate the main principles of this diet into your daily routine!

### A New Approach to Your Plate

Usually, you might decide on a protein around which to center your meal. Next, you add a couple of vegetable or starch dishes to go with this protein. Instead of this approach, try starting with one or two vegetables and making the protein an equal contributor, instead of the main event. It's not that you will be making more food; you will just need to approach the composition of the meal a little differently.

### Moderation is Essential

Regardless of the types of food you consume, it is essential to make sure you monitor the portion sizes. Portions are noticeably smaller within the Mediterranean diet, and the yields of the recipes in this book reflect that concept. You may be used to serving just four people with a pound of pasta, but you should try to stretch it to serve at least six. Additionally, a piece of chicken or meat for one person should be around five ounces.

Sorry, but you are not likely to encounter a 10-ounce steak on this diet! A Mediterranean lunch or dinner is made up of appropriately-sized contributions from a few different dishes.

## Eating Fresh and Local Foods

Much of Mediterranean meal planning focuses on maximizing vegetable and fruit consumption. Additionally, participants in this way of life celebrate seasonality by purchasing the product that is in season. Sticking to in-season produce helps you ensure that you get the freshest products possible. There are some canned and frozen versions of vegetables available year-round, of course. These include canned fava beans, frozen corn, canned tomatoes, and jarred artichoke hearts.

You'll find very little processed food on this diet. What you will discover are far more flavor and far fewer preservatives and sodium. Many of the dishes are brought to life by using herbs and spices instead of other, not-so-good-for-you ingredients. This diet is thousands of years old, dating to a time when you couldn't find all types of fruits and vegetables available 365 days a year like you can today. People ate what was in season. This practice is excellent because in-season produce has more nutrients than when it's out of season.

Buying local products also helps ensure you get the freshest ingredients. Fruits and vegetables lose nutrients the longer they sit in the refrigerator, so buying from local growers lets you know what you're getting is freshly picked and still contains many beneficial nutrients. But when fresh isn't available, people along the Mediterranean have learned to preserve food without using high amounts of salt, sugar, or fat, by drying beans and grains and drying and pickling vegetables.

Another key to the Mediterranean diet is that although about 35 percent of your caloric intake comes from fat, it is from *monounsaturated fats* – or healthy fats from olive oil, nuts, avocados, and fish. Nuts are a large part of the Mediterranean diet and contribute to your protein intake as well. Incorporating a handful of nuts every day can help boost your protein, omega-3 fatty acids, good fats, vitamin E, and fiber while reducing cholesterol.

## Daily Consumption of Whole Grains and Beans

Since Mediterranean inhabitants eat red meat and poultry sparingly, their major sources of protein include beans, lentils, nuts, and whole grains. These components can be featured in soups, stews, and salads. They also round out more filling dishes when combined with a source of protein, like fish. Additionally, they can enhance dishes that feature pasta or vegetables. Whole grains contribute many essential nutrients like antioxidants, but not all Mediterranean grains are whole grains.

## Consume Less Red Meat and More Seafood

The consumption of fresh fish and shellfish, has been a way of life in the countries along the Mediterranean Sea since men first started casting their fishing nets in that body of water. The benefits of eating seafood include their low-calorie count and high levels of heart-healthy polyunsaturated fats. Sardines and mackerel are included in the more affordable types of fresh fish. Fish can be prepared in many healthy ways including pan-roasting, broiling, grilling, and baking.

## Using Meat for Flavoring

Since red meat is typically expensive, it has been a common practice in the Mediterranean region to combine it with more economical ingredients, like beans or grains. That way, less meat is used overall. Those who practice this diet as a way of life implement this idea by creating dishes that highlight meat along with a central vegetable or grain. They may make use of more flavorful cuts of meat, so even a small portion of meat has an impressive effect.

### Serving Fruit for Dessert Instead of Sweets

Throughout the Mediterranean, fruit is often served as a dessert. Cakes and cookies are only eaten during special occasions, not every day. To try and lower the amount of saturated fat when you do serve sweets, you can try replacing all or part of the butter in your desserts with olive oil. Sometimes, to still produce a satisfying sweet that is worthy of serving to guests, you will need to keep some of the butter in the recipe. This idea may require you to do some experimentation as you endeavor to pursue this healthier way of eating and living.

### Variety is the Spice of Life

Mediterranean meals are full of diversity, so try serving dishes with a range of different temperatures and flavors. The idea of serving some foods cold helps make meal planning easier since some things can be made in advance or even served as leftovers. As you discover more and more dishes that fit into this eating plan, you'll find it is easy to mix and match recipes.

# The Mediterranean Diet Pyramid

In the 1990s cooperative work between nonprofit health and cultural food organization called ''Oldways'', and the Harvard School of Medicine led to a visual representation of the diet. This image was the 1993 creation of the Mediterranean Diet Pyramid. The visual representation of this way of eating serves as a handy tool for anyone interested in trying the diet. It essentially symbolized the results of the Seven Countries Study by Ancel Keys. One of his most important findings was that people who lived on the island of Crete, had lower rates of heart disease than the other study participants. Keys attributed this fact to their diet, which was full of vegetables, grains, and legumes and simultaneously low in saturated fat. The

Mediterranean Diet Pyramid ultimately helped make the diet popular in the United States. In 2008 the Mediterranean diet pyramid received some minor updates, and the result is the version described here.

Like the old USDA food pyramid of the 1990s, the Mediterranean Diet Pyramid places different types of foods in differently-sized spaces which represent their relative importance in this eating plan. The most common elements of Mediterranean meals, along with the plant products, form the base of the Pyramid. These include herbs and spices, nuts, olive oil, fruits and vegetables, whole grains, legumes, and beans. It is recommended that people following this diet base every meal on the foods in this large bottom space.

On the next level Pyramid, you will find seafood. Fish and shellfish should be consumed at least twice weekly. Further up are poultry and eggs, along with dairy products. These foods are eaten moderately in daily or weekly servings. At the very tip of the Mediterranean Pyramid are red meats and sweets, which are consumed in relatively small quantities and least often.

Off to the side of the Pyramid (or, in some versions, occupying a small space under meats and sweets) is red wine, which is safe to consume in moderation under this eating plan. When it comes to red wine, "moderation" generally means no more than one to two (5-ounce) glasses each day.

Additionally, the Pyramid contains a side reminder to hydrate by drinking plenty of water. You don't often see water in a food pyramid, but it's an integral part of any diet and lifestyle. More than half of your body is composed of water, making it a very integral part of nutrition. Drinking water is an important habit to develop as you exercise, too, because it helps boost your metabolism. You should focus on drinking plain water instead of sodas or sugary fruit drinks that could be filled with high fructose corn syrup. If you struggle with drinking enough plain water, try adding some fresh fruit or herbs to your glass to change the flavor.

Finally, in most versions of the Pyramid, another base piece consists of the essential components of the Mediterranean lifestyle: daily exercise, enjoying meals with others, relaxation, and smoking cessation.

## Recommended Servings and Serving Sizes

Although the Mediterranean diet pyramid doesn't go into a lot of details about how many servings and the serving sizes of each food group are recommended, there are some guidelines that dietary experts can agree on. The following guidelines should help you get an idea of how much of each food group in this diet you should try to eat, and what constitutes a serving size:

- **Whole Grains**: Four to six servings recommended each day.
   *Serving Size:* ½ cup cooked grains such as oats, quinoa, or pasta, or 1 slice of bread.
- **Vegetables:** Four to eight servings recommended each day.
   *Serving Size:* 1 cup raw or ½ cup cooked veggies.
- **Fruits:** Two to four servings recommended per day.
   *Serving Size:* ½ cup of fresh fruit or 1 average piece of fruit or ¼ cup dried fruit.
- **Beans and legumes:** One to three servings recommended each day.
   *Serving Size:* 1/3 cup dried or 1 cup cooked.
- **Seafood:** Two to three servings recommended each week.
   *Serving Size:* 4 to 6 ounces.

- **Fats:** Three to six servings recommended each day.
  *Serving Size:* 1 ounce of nuts or seeds (the number of nuts in an ounce depends on the size) or 2 tablespoons of groundnut or seed butter. For oils, a serving size is one tablespoon.
- **Herbs/Spices/Condiments:** Herbs can be used in large quantities. For condiments, aim for one tablespoon per serving. Salt should be reduced to 1 to 2 teaspoons per day.
- **Poultry:** One to three servings recommended each week.
  *Serving Size:* 3 to 4 ounces (should fit in the palm of your hand).
- **Red Meat:** No more than three to four servings recommended each month.
  *Serving Size:* 3 ounces
- **Eggs:** Three to four servings recommended per week (but egg whites can be eaten daily).
  *Serving Size:* 1 whole egg

- **Dairy:** One to three servings recommended per day.
  *Serving Size:* 1 cup of yogurt or 1 ounce of cheese; aim for low-fat or nonfat versions.
- **Alcohol:** Aim for no more than one to two drinks per day.
  *Serving Size:* 4 ounces of wine or 12 ounces of beer.
- **Sweets:** Avoid these and try to opt for one serving of fruit instead of other sugars.

In the case of the food groups in which a range of servings is recommended, use your common sense about your body size and activity level. If you are a tall, muscular person who gets a lot of physical activity, you can probably aim for the upper limits of serving sizes. For example, you could probably safely eat three servings of dairy per day, four servings of red meat per week, and six servings of healthy fats per day. Conversely, if you are a small or inactive person, or if your goal is to lose weight, you should try to eat the lower number of servings recommended for each food group. For more information about weight loss, see Chapter 5: "The Mediterranean Diet and Weight Loss.

# Chapter 3: Who Should Consider the Mediterranean Diet and Why?

This chapter delves into the Mediterranean Diet's many health benefits. If you find that you are attracted to these benefits or discover that it may be suitable for a specific health problem you currently face, you should certainly speak with your physician about adopting this eating plan.

Let's start by looking at the main parts of the Mediterranean Diet and their primary health benefits!

## The Main Parts and Health Benefits of the Mediterranean Diet

### Whole Grains

Whole grains are a vital part of the Mediterranean diet, and research has shown that consuming them decreases the risk of deadly diseases like diabetes and cancer, not to mention heart disease. A single whole grain kernel consists of an outer layer, called the bran (containing fiber); a middle layer (containing complex carbohydrates and protein); and an inner layer (including vitamins, minerals, and protein). Refining grains, a process that is common in the United States, leaves only the middle layer of the grain. This destruction of the most nutritious layers results in grains that do not have the vitamins and fiber known for fighting diseases. A few examples of whole grains you might use on this eating plan are kasha, barley, oatmeal, and farro.

Full of fiber, vitamins, minerals, and complex carbohydrates, whole grains present your body with numerous benefits. They aid digestion; decrease cholesterol levels, assist with weight loss because they keep you full longer; and help prevent deadly chronic diseases that are associated with poor cardiovascular health and high blood sugar. Whole grains are essential to people who have diabetes because they help regulate blood insulin levels.

### Fresh Fruits and Vegetables

Farmers' Markets in the Mediterranean region are typically full of fresh, in-season, locally-sourced fruits and vegetables. These natural foods contain high levels of vitamins, minerals, complex carbohydrates, and fiber that reduce the risk of cancer and heart disease, among other ailments. Phytonutrients, which are found at high levels under the skins of these plant products, are strong components that help us fight life-threatening health issues.

Fruits are easy to incorporate into your daily diet plan. You can buy fruit that's easily transportable, like apples, bananas, peaches, or apricots. Dried fruit is another great option. It's easy to pack and take with you, it won't spoil, it has an intense flavor, and most of the nutrients are retained. Fruits are also a great addition to your meals. Try adding dried fruit or pomegranate to salads, enhance the flavor of chicken with figs or dates, or add fresh fruit to a cup of Greek yogurt for a snack filled with protein and nutrients!

Fruits also contain natural sugars, which are easier for your body to digest and provide more nutrients than refined sugars. Natural sugars found in fruits are often called fructose. Although you've been trained to fear the word "sugar" and associate it with something terrible, naturally occurring sugars are essential for the body.

Now for vegetables. These good-for-you foods are another cornerstone of the Mediterranean diet. Vegetables are full of fiber, vitamins, minerals, chlorophyll, potassium, carotenoids, flavonoids, and antioxidants. They're also low in fat, sodium, and cholesterol. With the Mediterranean diet, vegetables should be at the base of every meal and should take up half your plate. They are very low in calories, so eating a lot of vegetables can be very beneficial – they'll fill you up with all the right nutrients, with nothing extra!

## Nuts

These tasty little morsels, like walnuts, pine nuts, and almonds, are full of heart-healthy monounsaturated fat, and they have long been a vital component of the Mediterranean diet. Because of their high fiber and protein level, nuts can help people lose weight because they help people who eat them to feel full for longer periods. They are also good sources of several key vitamins. Research has shown that eating nuts regularly is linked to lower risks of heart disease and heart attack and to lower cholesterol levels. Plus, nuts' fiber and antioxidants help your digestive system and slow cell aging.

However, nuts are high in calories, so eat in moderation. A handful a day can go a long way. Also, in a way, nuts are like vegetables: if you douse them with salt, sugar, and chocolate, you end up losing all the benefits they offer. So, skip the add-ons, and reap the rewards!

## Beans (Legumes)

Beans are also consumed regularly as a part of this diet. They contain high levels of fiber, which increase satiety and reduce cholesterol levels. Beans are also important sources of protein and vitamins. The fiber associated with regular bean consumption has been linked with a lowered risk of life-threatening issues like heart disease, cancer, and diabetes.

## Fish

Oily fish, prevalent in the Mediterranean diet, provide us with essential protein and omega-3 fatty acids. Omega-3 fatty acids have a favorable impact on cholesterol and triglyceride levels and help lower our risk of heart attack. They also help to reduce inflammation and, with regular consumption, decrease the risk of sudden death due to fatal cardiac arrhythmias.

The two omega-3 fatty acid types that you may have heard of in fish are *EPA (eicosapentaenoic acid)* and *DHA (docosahexaenoic acid)*. EPA is a fatty acid that prevents blood clotting and helps reduce pain and swelling. Its presence in your diet helps regulate and avoid issues like heart disease, Alzheimer's disease, personality disorders, depression, high blood pressure, and diabetes. DHA improves brain function, helps thin blood, and lowers triglyceride levels. It also reduces the risk of type 2 diabetes, heart disease, neurodegenerative diseases like dementia, and attention deficit hyperactivity disorder (ADHD).

A warning about fish: Several species of fish may contain high levels of mercury, and other contaminants, so pregnant women and young children should be careful. However, for most adults, the heart health benefits of fish consumption are much greater than the risks. To minimalize any risks, look for fish that contain the lowest mercury levels. The best choices are salmon, albacore tuna, herring, sardines, shad, trout, flounder, and pollock. It is best to avoid swordfish, shark, king mackerel, and tilefish because they usually have the highest mercury content.

## Olive Oil

Olive oil, made directly from olives that have been crushed and pressed, is the heart and soul of this eating plan. It provides much of the rich and distinctive flavor from the Mediterranean region, and it contains seemingly endless nutritional benefits. This oil is monounsaturated fat, which means that it boosts cardiac health. It also contains polyphenols, antioxidants, and omega-3 fatty acids. These vitamins and minerals help lower cholesterol while reducing our chances of developing diseases like cancer, heart disease, arthritis, osteoporosis, and even type-2 diabetes.

Using olive oil regularly instead of butter or margarine helps reduce your risk of heart disease, inflammatory disorders, cancer, and diabetes. Consuming olive oil also helps lower levels of bad (LDL) cholesterol while keeping or improving healthy levels of good (HDL) cholesterol.

Olive oil can assist with weight loss. A Boston study demonstrated that an eating plan that included regular consumption of nuts and olive oil led to sustained weight loss over a year and a half. This eating plan was compared to a low-fat diet. People also stayed on this olive oil- and nut-rich diet for a longer time because of these foods' satiety.

**Red Wine**

Moderate alcohol consumption has been shown to help reduce our risk of developing heart disease. Red wine in particular, often part of a Mediterranean meal, is believed to have several advantages over other forms of alcohol. Red wine consists of polyphenols and resveratrol, both of which promote cardiac health. Resveratrol is an antioxidant that helps maintain healthy levels of cholesterol and also contributes positively to blood clotting. It is present in higher levels in red wine than white.

It's critical to remember that alcohol should only be consumed in moderation. A person's daily wine consumption should not exceed one or two (5-ounce) glasses per day. For people who prefer to avoid wine, grape juice is an excellent alternative. Grape juice – specifically purple grape juice – also significantly reduces the risk of heart attack.

# Target Health Conditions of this Diet

You likely picked up on several health conditions that may receive benefits from components of the Mediterranean diet, but not all of them were included in previous descriptions. Below is a list of diseases or health conditions that can be improved or prevented by following a Mediterranean-based eating plan:

- Cancer
- Depression
- Dementia
- Diabetes
- High Blood Pressure/Stroke
- Heart Disease
- Metabolic Syndrome
- Obesity

## Focusing on Heart Disease

Many books and experts who talk about the Mediterranean diet focus almost exclusively on its benefits in heart disease prevention and overall contributions to heart health. The reason for this focus is simply that cardiovascular disease is the number one killer worldwide. Here's a rough breakdown of the eight most common ways people died in 2010 in the U.S.:

- Heart disease:                              600,000 deaths
- Cancer:                                     575,000 deaths
- Recurring lower respiratory diseases:       140,000 deaths
- Stroke:                                     130,000 deaths

- Accidents: 120,000 deaths
- Alzheimer's disease: 85,000 deaths
- Diabetes: 70,000 deaths
- Kidney disease: 50,000 deaths

At a glance, heart disease and cancer death seem comparable. However, when you look at deaths caused by cardiovascular disease – which is responsible for heart disease but also affects the entire circulatory system – they number more than 800,000. This includes heart disease, stroke (90 percent are the clotting type related to the very same process that causes heart attacks), and many other blood-vessel-related conditions. Diabetes, Alzheimer, and kidney disease are also thought to be linked to or worsened by cardiovascular disease. Cancer is number two on the list, resulting in around 575,000 deaths. However, of those, 160,000 cases are lung cancer, in which the majority are related to smoking. The next most common cancers are colorectal (50,000 deaths per year), breast (40,000), pancreatic (40,000), and prostate (30,000). Each one of these cancers can be caused by a combination of many different factors – such as genetics, diet, environmental toxins, hormones, and various other carcinogens. Cardiovascular disease, in contrast, has a more unified cause, so following its prevention plan has the potential the help most people's greatest risk. Furthermore, the same diet and lifestyle recommendations that help prevent heart and cardiovascular disease generally help protect from cancer – and all the other major chronic diseases – as well.

# A History of Research Behind the Mediterranean Diet

The pursuit of an ideal diet began in earnest when heart attacks began increasing at an alarming rate in the 1940s. No health concern was more urgent than heart disease at that time, as it was responsible for around 40 percent of the total deaths in the United States (and if you included stroke, which is related to the same disease process, the figure was 50 percent). The overall death rate was much higher then as well, and a disease of the arteries caused about half the deaths. Again and again, men and women in the prime of life were dropping from sudden cardiac death. It wasn't long before the leader of the United States, President Dwight Eisenhower, had a massive heart attack at the age of 65, while still in office. The nation was on edge and looking for answers.

Evidence that the Mediterranean way of eating can be beneficial to people who suffer from cardiovascular disease, and other conditions was ultimately discovered in some independent and widely-publicized research projects and clinical trials. Here, we'll look at some of them:

## The Seven Countries Study

Previously mentioned in the description of the Mediterranean Food Pyramid, this landmark twenty-year study by Dr. Ancel Keys was able to show that a diet that contained low levels of saturated animal fat and processed food was linked to a low incidence in mortality from coronary heart disease and cancer. Diet had been suggested as a probable cause for heart disease since at least the turn of the century, but an understanding of the connection remained murky at this point. Cholesterol had been identified as a likely candidate for having something to do with it, singled out because it was found that the arterial clots themselves were full of it. When some substantial studies came out demonstrating that cholesterol levels in the blood were higher in patients with heart disease, many thought they had at last confirmed the dietary culprit. However, Keys performed studies that showed it was not the cholesterol one *ate* that made it available in the blood to form blockages in the arteries.

Keys had begun to hypothesize what else it might be other than cholesterol in the diet that was causing those high levels when an unusual patient took him in a new direction. A sick farmer was referred to him by a medical school in Wisconsin. After trying various treatments, Keys checked the farmer's blood cholesterol level, and the first reading was sky high – 1,000 mg/dL, compared with the national average of 220 or 230. The man's brother had come in with him as well and had a reading of 600. The two were sent to Keys' Minnesota lab, where they stayed and were fed an almost fat-free diet for a week. After a week, their cholesterol levels had both dropped by about 50 percent. Keys wondered what might happen if he gave them some fat. When he gave them food with saturated fat in it, the cholesterol levels of both men increased dramatically. Hence, it appeared that it was *fat* that was affecting their cholesterol levels. It was ultimately the result of this particular investigation that led to his painstaking testing of how fats, in their many forms, could affect health and disease.

Keys went on to perform further feeding studies, which convinced him that, indeed, blood cholesterol levels were the result of how much fat was consumed in the diet. Postwar statistics also revealed an intriguing clue to the mystery. Keys noticed that some of the wealthiest, and probably best-fed, people in America suffered from significantly high incidences of heart disease. However, in postwar Europe, where supplies of food like meat and dairy were quite low, heart disease rates had declined. He was also impressed and intrigued by the alleged low rates of heart disease being reported in the area around the

Mediterranean Sea. Ultimately, upon invitation from an Italian colleague, he left for Italy in 1952.

From a research standpoint, Keys' stay in Italy was the dawn of collecting international health and nutritional data to compare with other regions. For example, it quickly became clear to him that cholesterol levels in Naples were much lower than those being measured in America and England. It also soon became clear as he toured Italian hospitals that heart disease in this region was indeed a rarity. From here, Keys continued to expand his research, collecting data from Madrid, Spain as well. His reports stimulated an international group to join in, generating measurements and diagnoses in South Africa, Japan, and Finland.

The collective data supported the notion that differing fats in the diet were associated with varying blood cholesterol levels, as well as in the frequency of heart disease. In Japan, for example, they observed communities with a low incidence of heart disease who ate a very low-fat diet, whereas in Finland they encountered hard-working men, many of whom were quite physically fit by outward appearances. However, in this land of butter and cheese, many of these apparently fit men suffered from heart disease.

Keys observed and followed the lifestyle patterns in Naples, where he was staying. He became enamored with the food and culture of southern Italy. Keys absorbed and embraced the people's culinary tastes and habits, their tendency to walk everywhere and get out in the sunshine, their tendency to drink a glass or two of wine with supper. This seaside introduction to the culture of Naples turned out to be just as important as the scientific revelations to come. He found that the diet of this region was loaded with fruits, vegetables, and whole grains. The way of eating here was also different from certain other diets in that it contained significantly fewer dairy and meat products and offered fewer sweet baked goods for dessert. These observations culminated in his development of the Seven Countries Study.

With the active participation of leading international cardiologist Paul Dudley White (President Eisenhower's cardiologist), the study was a meticulously planned and executed ten-year investigation of the epidemiology of coronary disease in sixteen populations of six Western countries and Japan. Around 13,000 men were studied, aged forty to fifty-nine, from Japan, Greece, the Netherlands, Finland, Yugoslavia (formerly), Greece, and Italy. It took years of negotiations, fundraising, planning, and trial run before communities began being monitored in 1958. This massive endeavor was a milestone study on numerous counts, marking the first effort in history to leap international borders and compare diet-disease associations between communities with widely differing culinary and lifestyle populations. The hope was that the regional differences in risk, health behavior, and biological factors could be measured, thus providing direction to prevent – or at the very least decelerate – heart disease around the world.

The first results from the Seven Countries Study were published in 1970, after ten years of data collecting. As Keys had predicted, a high amount of fat in the diet – especially saturated fat – was correlated with heart disease. Both the island of Crete in Greece and southern Italy were heralded as the shining stars of the study, having by far the lowest proportion of heart disease and the longest life expectancy. Americans, by contrast, had a 72 percent greater chance of dying from heart disease than the Italians. It was clear that diet was related, but since only the macronutrient contents were used for analysis (that is, the amounts of proteins, carbohydrates, and fats), the specific foods of the diets were not published for some time.

33

The Seven Countries Study generated much interest in the eating habits of the healthiest people in the world. Over time, more research was published that demonstrated the benefits for the other elements of the Mediterranean diet aside from eating little saturated fat. It turned out that all the antioxidants, vitamins, minerals, fiber, healthy proteins, complex carbohydrates, and wine these people were consuming promoted health and longevity as well.

Throughout the 1980s and 1990s, scientists, nutritionists, and doctors worked to define what the Mediterranean diet precisely was. After all, there are more than fifteen countries that surround the Mediterranean Sea, with overlapping cuisines. Which formula was the best? In the end, they kept coming back to the 1960s rural diets of Crete and southern Italy. Also, in 1989, one of the directors involved in the Seven Countries Study published a historical record of what the subjects in all the countries under investigation were eating around the time of the study. The proportions for Crete and southern Italy at that time are now taken to be the ideal healthy Mediterranean diet, because of those communities' very low incidence of various diet-linked conditions (though their diets and disease rates have since changed). Other investigations confirmed the data and thus constituted the principal research basis for the proportions of foods in modern Mediterranean diet pyramids.

### The Lyon Diet Heart Study

One of the first clinical trials in support of the therapeutic benefits of the Mediterranean eating plan, a groundbreaking study known as the Lyon Diet Heart Study, came in 1994. Six hundred patients in France who had had heart attacks were randomly assigned to either a Mediterranean-style diet, or a control diet similar to what the American Heart Association recommended for the reduction of heart disease risk. Two years into the study, the compelling results came in: the Mediterranean group had a 73 percent reduced risk of coronary events, and 70 percent reduced overall chance of dying as compared with the control diet. The study was meant to go for five years but was stopped after an interim analysis showed such significant beneficial effects in the patients receiving the Mediterranean diet. Adding to the significance of this study was the intriguing finding that, despite a robust connection between adhering to the Mediterranean diet and living longer, no significant associations were seen for the individual components of the diet. It was becoming clear that it was the diet as a whole that was best for your overall health, and protection from disease.

As research continued, it also became apparent that the Mediterranean diet was not just better for your heart. Any condition related to arteries or veins generally benefitted. Data from a series of studies have also shown that sticking to the Mediterranean diet is can help lower the risk of developing various cancers. The risk of contracting degenerative diseases of the brain such as Parkinson's and Alzheimer's appears to be cut as well. Moreover, the Mediterranean diet has long been recognized to reduce mortality overall.

Below is a summary of several other scientific investigations that contributed to the evidence pointing to the Mediterranean diet's myriad health benefits:

## The DART Study

In this research project, over 2,000 men were studied to test whether the polyunsaturated fat in seafood would help protect against heart disease. The results showed that eating a modest serving of oily fish twice per week reduced the risk of heart disease death by 32 percent and overall mortality by 29 percent.

### The Alzheimer's Disease Study

Dr. Nikolaos Scarmeas, from New York's Columbia University Medical Center, showed that a Mediterranean diet was linked to a 68 percent lower chance of developing Alzheimer's disease. He led another study that demonstrated that eating a Mediterranean food helped Alzheimer's disease patients to live longer, healthier lives even after their initial diagnosis.

### The Singh Indo-Mediterranean Diet Study

This trial placed 499 patients who were at risk for heart disease on a diet that was full of foods derived from plants. The study found that the diet change reduced incidences of heart attack and sudden cardiac death. Researchers also discovered that the subjects had fewer cardiovascular events, overall than those on a conventional diet.

### The Metabolic Syndrome Study

Dr. Katherine Esposito and her Italian colleagues tested the effects of a Mediterranean diet on patients who suffered from metabolic syndrome (a condition that is characterized by obesity, elevated blood pressure, unhealthy cholesterol profile, and indications of vascular inflammation). The Mediterranean diet improved all the symptoms of metabolic syndrome.

### The Spain Study

This Spanish study compared a Mediterranean diet to a diet that was low in fat. Although planned for a longer period the study abruptly ceased after just 4.8 years, because of the those following the Mediterranean diet showed a massive 30 percent reduction in significant cardiovascular incidents (i.e., heart attack, stroke, death). In the *New York Times* on March 2, 2013, medical experts stated that for the first time in history a diet had been proven to be as effective as drugs in preventing cardiovascular complications, including death.

## Recent Thoughts About the Mediterranean Diet

By the year 2000, the quantity of fat in the Mediterranean diet came under scrutiny, challenging many deeply held beliefs that a low-fat diet was the ideal. It was acknowledged that, even though high amounts of fat in the diet were linked to heart disease, some of the regions the Mediterranean diet were modeled after actually had a high-fat content in their food, up to around 40 percent of their daily calories. But it wasn't saturated fat they had been eating – their diet had olive oil poured all over it. With a combination of monounsaturated fat and antioxidants that benefit health in numerous ways, olive oil seemed to be an essential health elixir, helping to thwart disease in many shapes and forms.

An interdisciplinary, multicultural conference was held in Rome to further update and standardize the Mediterranean diet in 2005. The participants invoked an ancient Greek word, *ataraxia* – which connotes "equilibrium," "lifestyle," and being in a state of robust tranquility while surrounded with trustworthy and affectionate friends – to accompany the description of the Mediterranean diet. In presenting it as more than just a diet, they recognized the importance of the entire lifestyle upon health and well-being. Physical, social, and culinary activities also play an essential role.

Unfortunately, scientists still have not found a magic bullet for health, probably because one does not exist – our bodies are far too complicated for that. However, at this point, we seem to have identified the diet of the people who have the least disease and live the longest. Perhaps the magic is that the Mediterranean diet improves universal biological features that promote health, such as reducing inflammation and excess body fat; maybe it's the environment of warm social connection enjoyed by the healthiest communities; maybe it's that a diet so fresh, varied, and delicious, yet simple, is so easy to take on. It is most certainly partly all these things.

## Who Should Consider Switching to the Mediterranean Diet?

The answer to this question seems pretty straightforward. Anyone who wishes to pursue ideal cardiovascular health and consequently do all they can to prevent death by diet- or lifestyle-related complications should consider the Mediterranean diet! In other words, experts have presented a strong case for the idea that this eating plan is ideal for just about anyone!

### Possible Socioeconomic Limitations

However, research published in 2017 showed that the benefits of this diet might be limited to people of higher income status, higher socioeconomic backgrounds, or who are more "educated". Specifically, researchers found that advantages to heart health from the Mediterranean diet may be limited to only top socioeconomic status groups.

The reasons behind these findings could be several different things. First, it is possible that the higher quality of food available to the upper socioeconomic classes is responsible for the benefits of this diet. Additionally, a more extensive variety of food is available to those at a higher income level. Finally, it is highly possible that those with more education were able to adhere to the diet more closely and recall their adherence with better accuracy. In other words, perhaps not everyone reported their strict following of the menu with perfect recall. Because many possible details that influence how well people report their eating habits, this research is not necessarily accurate or reliable.

Does this study mean that those of us who earn lower incomes or did not pursue education after high school, should throw up our hands and give up all hope of benefitting from a Mediterranean diet? Of course not! It just means that everyone, regardless of income, background, or education level, needs to commit firmly to the eating plan if they wish to reap its rewards. No one is expecting perfection, but what matters is that we all make small and continual strides towards improvement.

Additionally, it is possible that those of us who earn lower incomes may face more significant challenges when it comes to finding high-quality ingredients. However, it is possible to follow the Mediterranean diet on a limited budget. In general, whole, unprocessed foods are more affordable than their more processed counterparts. Fresh fruits and vegetables, especially when locally sourced, are usually economical. Canned light tuna in water has just as many health benefits as fresh salmon. There are many affordable whole grains, and poultry is generally budget-friendly. Since red meat and dairy are eaten in limited quantities, these items should not impact your bank account too much.

As far as more expensive items, like olive oil, herbs, and spices go, it is suggested that you purchase these things in limited quantities anyway. If you have too much of any of these items on hand, you run the risk of them spoiling before you can use them. In the next chapter, you'll see the most commonly used spices and herbs, so you'll get an idea of where to start. Additionally, it is suggested that you start with just what you need for the first few recipes you plan to make, and then build slowly from there. There is also a buying guide for olive oil!

**Those with Food Allergies and Sensitivities**

It is true that the Mediterranean diet includes several components that are highly allergenic to some people, including certain nuts, shellfish, dairy, and products that contain gluten. However, even those people can follow this eating plan with a few adjustments!

For those who are allergic to shellfish, dairy, or nuts, there are plenty of options for protein and unsaturated fats in this diet, so you should be able to follow it while making the necessary substitutions. You have likely already become accustomed to making these changes in your diet, so these adjustments are not likely to be very difficult for you.

For people who have gluten allergies or sensitivities, there is no reason that you cannot follow this diet as well. Those who have not researched the Mediterranean diet sometimes incorrectly assume that it is full of bread and pasta. However, at this point in the book, you should understand that there are many other integral parts to this diet which do not contain any wheat or gluten whatsoever. Additionally, many whole grains do not contain gluten, like the following: amaranth, buckwheat, corn, millet, most whole oats, rice, sorghum, and wild rice.

Also, quinoa, although technically not a grain, can be consumed similarly to grain, and it does not contain gluten. If you have been diagnosed with gluten intolerance, like Krone's disease, or gluten sensitivity, you are likely already used to making gluten-free substitutions and adjustments to your diet. You can rest assured that the Mediterranean diet is not off-limits to you!

**REMINDER: Always Consult Your Doctor!**

Regardless of your physical fitness, health concerns, or food allergies, it is always strongly recommended that you consult your healthcare provider before changing diets or beginning a new exercise program. Your doctor can address any underlying concerns that may make it necessary for you to pursue a particular variation of the Mediterranean diet. He may recommend that you undergo specific testing before making any dietary changes or after following a new diet for several months.

In the next chapter, you'll learn how to start making the necessary steps towards incorporating the Mediterranean diet and mindset into your lifestyle.

# Chapter 4: Getting Started

Changing your eating habits to follow the Mediterranean diet can be very exciting. Knowing that you're making the conscious decision to improve your diet – and your life – in a positive way and eat healthier is the first step of the Mediterranean diet. It might seem overwhelming at first, but you don't have to make all the changes in one day. The more small changes you make, the more benefits you'll see, which will inspire you to make more beneficial changes. Those benefits will pay off big in the long run – for you and your family.

## Keys to Embracing the Mediterranean Lifestyle

To successfully incorporate this new way of eating into your life, you should seriously consider adopting other parts of the Mediterranean lifestyle as well.

### Reduce Your Stress Level

Remember the discussion of the dangers of stress in Chapter 1? One of the most critical keys to revamping your lifestyle to fit your new way of eating is *stress reduction*! This instruction may be a tricky one; after all, we all have periods of stress in our lives. Additionally, some of us seem destined to have more pressure in our lives than other people. Regardless, handling stress should begin with trying to find a realistic perspective on the factors that cause our stress, then doing what we can to change those factors. Maybe you can't really follow the Mediterranean habit of taking a 2-hour midday break, but you can incorporate ways to reduce your stress throughout your day.

First, a physical exercise program will help tremendously in stress reduction, simply because research has shown that active people can handle pressure better. There is an explanation for the beneficial effects of exercise on stress levels: People who engage in regular aerobic exercise have lower adrenaline levels that rise less dramatically in stressful situations.

Try to get some physical activity every day. It can be something as casual as walking your children to the park or walking your dog for 20 minutes while enjoying nature instead of looking at your phone. If you can't do something physical, try preparing a cup of coffee or tea, disconnecting from technology, and sitting on your porch to relax and sip it for 20 minutes. It's the little things that allow your body and mind to rest.

In addition to a regular exercise program, some form of relaxation practice such as meditation, yoga, or self-hypnosis can also help reduce your overall stress level. If all these lifestyle changes do not result in a significant reduction in stress, then consider a consultation with a psychologist or psychiatrist.

Below are ten practices for you to try for stress reduction:

- Daily exercise
- Meditation
- Prayer
- Enjoying close relationships with friends and family
- Setting realistic goals in life
- Living within your (financial) means
- Yoga
- Enjoying interests and hobbies outside of work
- Having an optimistic outlook on life and never losing your sense of humor
- Laughing, smiling, and enjoying your life!

**Exercise Daily**

Although this recommendation was mentioned under stress reduction, it bears further investigation. Daily exercise is a very important part of the Mediterranean lifestyle, and it does more than help you handle stress. Whether it's walking to the market or working in the garden (two common forms of daily exercise in the Mediterranean region), regular daily exercise is essential for good health. Activity raises good (HDL) cholesterol, lowers blood pressure and optimizes bone health, which reduces the risk of osteoporosis. Regular exercise also promotes a healthy sense of well-being; no wonder why there are so many healthy and happy senior citizens in the Mediterranean region of the world!

Lack of exercise, along with poor food choices, has contributed to the recent outbreak of American obesity. Additionally, several studies have shown that being out of shape physically is more detrimental to our health than just being overweight. Sadly, we have become a nation of "couch potatoes," and getting people to adopt a habit of exercising is difficult. We like using the elevator instead of the stairs; we park as close as possible to the store; we ride in carts instead of walking through a nine-or-18-hole game of golf!

The solution is to begin incorporating exercise into your daily activities. You do not need to start with anything ridiculous by jogging 5 miles a day or biking for an hour every morning. Just walking for thirty minutes a day can significantly decrease the risk of heart attack or other cardiovascular problems. Additionally, a regular exercise program will reduce fatigue and improve your lung function. If you add resistance training with light weights, your bone health will improve further, and you'll be helping to maintain your muscle tone.

It's up to you to decide what physical activity you enjoy, figure out how you can make it a part of your life, and stick with it until it becomes a habit. You can integrate many different forms of exercise into your daily life. Among of which are walking during your lunch break, walking the kids to the park instead of driving, going for a bike ride on Saturday morning instead of watching cartoons, walking between stores instead of driving when you're out shopping, or playing a sport the entire family can enjoy. If you have children, you can set an example that physical activity should be part of their lives as well.

Here are some more easy tips for incorporating exercise into your life:

- Walk in place for thirty minutes while watching TV.
- Park farther away from your office, grocery store, etc. and enjoy a short walk through the parking lot.
- Walk for the first part of your lunch break, before you eat.
- Use a pedometer and aim to get 10,000 steps each day.
- Choose to take the stairs for a change.

Physical activity is an indispensable part of the Mediterranean diet, and order to be successful with adopting this eating plan, you must integrate exercise into your life as well as making healthy eating choices.

**Family Time**

In the fast-paced and highly technical era we live in, it's sometimes hard to make time for family. However, it should be a priority. Try planning dinner times so everyone can sit and eat a meal together. It helps build relationships and connections. Much research has shown that people with strong family interaction are less likely to suffer from depression.

If you don't live near any family members, you can create the same atmosphere with friends. Try planning weekly or bi-weekly get-togethers and maybe having a different friend host it each time. Making meals potlucks takes the stress off any one person preparing a big meal. When you go, take a Mediterranean diet recipe to share with your friends!

## Other Tips for the Mediterranean Way of Life

Besides reducing your stress level, getting more daily physical activity, and increasing your family time, the following are solid guidelines that you should consider beginning to incorporate into your new way of life. Remember, no one is expecting you to make dramatic changes overnight. You can start each of these guidelines with baby steps, then work your way into more significant changes:

- Eat a variety of fresh, whole foods
- Limit intake of fat, except healthy sources of unsaturated fat
- Avoid refined sugar
- Avoid excessive salt
- Limit portion size
- Consume alcohol only in moderation (preferably red wine)
- Hydrate by drinking plenty of water!
- Laugh, smile, and enjoy life – never lose your sense of humor.
- No smoking! If you do smoke, take steps to begin quitting today.
- Relax a little every day (especially after meals, if possible)

# A Fresh Look at Your Kitchen

Stocking your kitchen is so important when adopting a new way of eating. You do not want to be left with a pantry empty of healthy foods, and only chips or a boxed cake mix as your meal or snack options. Keeping a well-stocked pantry gives you more alternatives and ideas of dishes you can make. Experimenting with different herbs, spices, and flavors is also important because these are low-calorie and fat-free ways of adding a tremendous amount of flavor to any dish, all completely guilt free.

While you will be using lots of familiar ingredients like chicken, salmon, quinoa, and chickpeas in the Mediterranean diet, you should also investigate less familiar ingredients and research recipes for grains like barley, beans like chickpeas, meats like oxtails, and fantastic seafood like monkfish. Depending on how in-depth you wish to pursue this way of eating and living, you may want to learn to work with finicky ingredients like grape leaves and phyllo dough and flavor builders like sumac, preserved lemons, and pomegranate molasses.

This book only has 20 recipes, which is just a small start to an infinite number of other equally-healthy dishes that you can find through research. Below is information about core kitchen ingredients you may want to begin stocking. It is not recommended that you buy all the spices, herbs, condiments, and other long-lasting ingredients at once. To do so would be extremely costly! Instead, decide on the recipes you want to try first, and begin your shopping list with the ingredients necessary for those dishes. Eventually, you'll find that your pantry and refrigerator are well-stocked with ingredients from each of the following categories:

## Fresh Fruits and Vegetables

Fruits and vegetables are a large portion of the Mediterranean diet food pyramid, so let's look at them first. When purchasing these foods, it's best to buy items that are in season, when they're at their peak flavor. Buying produce in season, and as close to the time it was picked, ensures you get fruits or vegetables with the most nutrients. One way to ensure you're getting fresh produce is to buy from local farms and farmers' markets. It's also a good idea to smell produce before you buy it. If it smells great, it's likely to taste great, too.

Here are some critical fruits in the Mediterranean diet: Apples, apricots, avocados, bananas, berries, dates, figs, grapes, melons, olives, peaches, pomegranate, and strawberries.

The following are some of the vegetables that are popular on this diet: Artichokes, beets, bell peppers, carrots, cauliflower, dandelion greens, eggplants, garlic, leafy greens, onions, potatoes, romaine lettuce, tomatoes, and zucchini.

You may have noticed that tomatoes are on the vegetable list. Technically, tomatoes are a fruit, not a vegetable. But because most people recognize them as a veggie and prepare them like they would other vegetables, they are listed with the other vegetables here. Tomatoes and tomato products are a huge part of the Mediterranean diet, from fresh tomatoes to tomato sauce, tomato paste, and so much more.

Many recipes in this book, and from the Mediterranean region, include garlic and onions. These two ingredients can provide an abundance of flavor to any dish. They're versatile and can be cooked in different ways to alter their flavors and pungency, too. For example, when onions are sautéed slowly, they give off a sweet taste, and when garlic is toasted in olive oil, it has a nutty flavor. Both can also be used raw atop a salad or in a dressing.

Also in the recipes, you'll see how often vegetables are easily integrated into the recipes and prepared in so many different ways. But remember that vegetables on their own are very healthy, so don't load them with heavy creams or sauces that add lots of calories and fat. And keep in mind that the more vegetables you eat, the more your body benefits. So work them into your meal plan as often as you can.

## Canned and Dried Beans

Legumes are an integral protein in the Mediterranean diet – in fact, they help make up the most extensive section of the menu, along with fruits, vegetables, and whole grains. Legumes can be eaten green or harvested and dried for their beans or seeds. This group includes chickpeas, fava beans, lentils, peas, and white beans. They can be eaten alone or also prepared as a part of a recipe with other ingredients. Two examples might be whole-wheat spaghetti with lentils or shrimp with white beans.

Canned beans typically work well in salads, sautés, and soups. You may consider using dried beans in recipes that take a longer time to cook, such as stews. In these dishes, cooking the beans can help develop the flavor more completely. Some people like to prepare dried beans by brining them; this preparation helps them to keep their original shape during the cooking process. Fava beans are one of the only beans that are more frequently used fresh than dried or canned, although preparing fresh fava beans is somewhat labor-intensive.

Legumes and their seeds are very inexpensive, and when dried, they last a long time. These ingredients are prevalent in Mediterranean countries because they store easily and can be used throughout the winter, when traditionally the availability of meat or vegetables was low. Rehydrating them is very simple – just soak in water for a few hours and cook as desired. You can also rehydrate them, cook them in water, and freeze the cooked legumes. Then, when you're craving hummus, you can just defrost the beans in minutes, rather than a few hours. Using dried beans is also a great alternative to using canned goods which can sometimes have many preservatives.

## Grains

Grains, including rice, are central to many Mediterranean dishes. There are different ways to cook each type of grain. For example, farro should be boiled in an excessive amount of water, but rice only needs just enough boiling water to absorb it all fully. You should strive to have at least 50 percent of the total grains you eat be whole grains. As mentioned previously in this guide, refined grains contain far fewer beneficial nutrients and can even negatively impact your risk of developing diseases like diabetes.

Some of the many examples of whole grains include bulgar, corn, oats, barley, brown rice, buckwheat, farro, freekeh, spelt, wheat berries, whole rye, whole-wheat flour, and wheatberries. Quinoa, although it is actually a nutty-flavored seed, can also be placed in this category because it's commonly thought of as a grain and is typically prepared and eaten in the same fashion as other grains.

Whole grains are incredibly versatile. You can use them in soups; prepare them as pilafs; work them into bread, cakes or cookies; or even use them as a stuffing. It's simple to make any dish a bit healthier by replacing all-purpose flour with whole-wheat flour, for example. Or replace long-grain rice with brown rice and regular pasta with whole-wheat pasta.

## Pasta and Couscous

Pasta is an essential part of many Mediterranean dishes, but it is frequently prepared in ways that are not familiar to most American home cooks. For example, some pasta dishes get their distinctive flavors from strong spices like cinnamon or cloves. Heartily robust whole-wheat pasta should be a nice change from the typical pasta to which most Americans are accustomed.

Couscous is commonly eaten in North Africa as a part of many diverse dishes, and it is sometimes served on its own. Residents of the eastern part of this region use a type of couscous called pearl couscous, which has larger grains and is toasted instead of dried.

## Olives and Olive Oil

Olives are quite well-known for their role in Mediterranean food. Many types are crushed and pressed to make olive oil, but others are grown exclusively for eating. If your grocery store has a refrigerated section with olives, those are more highly recommended than the canned and jarred types, since the preservatives in those make them very salty. If you have enough food preparation time, experts even suggest that you purchase olives that still have the pits, then remove the pits from them yourself.

You will learn more about olive oil in a different section of this chapter.

## Fresh and Dried Herbs

Herbs and spices were added to the pyramid representing the Mediterranean diet in 2008 because they are such an essential component of this diet. They add an abundance of flavor without extra calories or fat. They also add some vitamins and minerals to your diet. And they're long-lasting: dried herbs and spices often stay good for at least a year when stored in an airtight container.

Some recipes call for fresh herbs, while others call for dried. Why the difference? Flavor. The flavor of fresh herbs can be very earthy and pungent, while dried herbs are nuttier and toned down. You can add fresh herbs to recipes without needing to cook them, whereas dried herbs more than likely need to be prepared to bring out their flavor.

The dishes of the Mediterranean region are flavored by a wide variety of fresh herbs, such as basil and mint. Many proponents of this diet grow these herbs themselves, while other people purchase them from stores or farmer's markets. In the recipes of this book, fresh herbs are used as a garnish for some recipes, but they contribute to the main flavors of other dishes. Most fresh herbs will not last long in storage, but with proper handling, you should be able to keep them for a week or so. First, you'll need to rinse them carefully, then dry them as thoroughly and as gently as possible. Then roll them in paper towels, but keep the rolls loose. The last step is to place the roll of herbs and paper towels in a bag with a zipper seal and keep it in your refrigerator.

You should also strive to keep plenty of different dried herbs available because many Mediterranean recipes call for them. Blends of various herbs are a terrific way to add complex flavor to dishes. Dried herbs lose their flavor 12 or fewer months after you open the container. You can test them for their freshness by rubbing a pinch of one between your fingers. If you do not detect that herb's signature aroma, you should discard it and buy a new supply. Some herbs that you purchase fresh can be dried in the microwave, but this should only be attempted with the heartier herbs, like rosemary and thyme.

Here are some common herbs in the Mediterranean diet: Basil, bay leaf, cilantro, marjoram, mint, oregano, parsley, rosemary, sage, and thyme.

## Mediterranean Spices and Spice Blends

The various cuisines in the Mediterranean region can typically be distinguished from each other by the spices that are used in the recipes. You may already have some of the spices you'll need, like cinnamon and paprika. Other spices, like sumac and Aleppo pepper, will be less known to you. Spice pastes and dry blends are also frequently used to add distinctive flavors to dishes: Examples include *za'atar*, a favorite eastern Mediterranean blend; North African *ras el hanout*; and *harissa*, a North African chili paste. You can purchase these and other spice blends at some supermarkets or grocery stores, but if you are unable to find them at the store, you can learn to make your own with a little practice and research.

Storing your spices at a safe distance from heat and light will help you keep them longer. You should pay attention to the smell and appearance of each spice; when either of these characteristics changes, it's probably time to throw it out. When buying spices, you'll find that the better brands are usually pricier, but the difference it makes in your recipes is often well worth the extra cost. Additionally, a little spice goes a long way, so the price isn't so bad if you consider how many meals you can get out of one small bottle of any spice.

The following are common spices used in Mediterranean cooking: Allspice, black pepper, cayenne, cinnamon, cloves, coriander, cumin, dried ginger, paprika, sumac, and zaatar.

## Salt

Salt enables you to get the most flavor from a dish. That's why you'll see salt called for in almost every recipe in this book. You can use table salt, which is the most common type, or you can use sea salt instead if you like. Sea salt has more minerals and is an organic salt, while table salt, on the other hand, is more processed. And don't worry about the sodium content of these recipes. The tiny dashes of salt you'll be adding only increase the sodium minimally. The high levels of sodium that are detrimental to cardiovascular health, are found in processed foods that contain vast quantities of salt-laden preservatives to extend the shelf life of the product.

## Cheeses, Cured Meats, and Nuts

Just a little bit of cheese, like feta; cured meat, like pancetta; or nuts can add a lot of flavor to Mediterranean recipes. For example, some dishes are flavored with just a little bit of salami or prosciutto, while many kinds of pasta and salad dishes need only a tiny sprinkle of Parmesan cheese to round out their flavor.

Nuts are standard in the Mediterranean diet. They're tasty on their own or in many sweet or savory dishes. Whether roasted, toasted, or raw, walnuts, pine nuts, almonds, pistachios, sesame seeds, peanuts, cashews, and other nuts are full of flavor. They are frequent additions to salads and other side dishes. Additionally, some seasoning blends include nuts as an important component. Some of the recipes later in the book demonstrate how easily you can add nuts to your diet.

Although the recommended intake for dairy is only two servings per day, still opt for low-fat versions because dairy products are high in saturated fat. Avoid processed cheeses and instead choose fresh cheese made of sheep's or goat's milk. These are usually more flavorful, and a little goes a long way.

When you plan to store cheese in the refrigerator for more than a few days, you should wrap it first in parchment paper, which lets the cheese breathe. The top layer over the parchment paper should be aluminum foil. This impenetrable layer keeps the cheese from drying out and also keeps out unwanted flavors from other refrigerator inhabitants. For long-term storage of nuts, keep them in your freezer; otherwise, you run the risk of them becoming rancid. To bring out the flavor of nut in recipes, try toasting them in the microwave or on the stovetop before incorporating them into dishes.

## Fresh Meats, Poultry, Eggs, and Seafood

The Mediterranean diet includes many types of meats, including beef and lamb, poultry and eggs, and seafood, providing much-needed protein in small serving sizes.

Beef, lamb, and goat are conventional in the Mediterranean region, although they are eaten in limited quantities. When purchasing red meats, opt for the leanest cuts. Fillet, although it's costly, is an excellent cut of red meat because it's tender and very lean. You can grill it without adding any fat and can season with fresh or dried herbs and spices to enhance the flavor. For ground meat, whether it's beef or lamb, aim for 95 percent lean and 5 percent fat ground. The small amount of fat helps keep the meat moist and flavorful. Adding spices can also boost the flavor.

Poultry and eggs are other great sources of protein. Chicken, duck, turkey, and fowl are usually quite affordable and can be prepared in many different ways. To eliminate a lot of saturated fat when cooking poultry, remove the skin. And if you're looking for a piece of leaner meat, use the breast. The recommended portion of poultry is 1 (6- to 8-oz) serving every 2 days.

Over the years, eggs have developed an unfortunate reputation for being high in fat and cholesterol, but when you're on the Mediterranean diet, you should have no reason to avoid eggs. This eating plan recommends that you eat up to 7 eggs per week. They are a top source of high-quality protein and are still low in calories.

Seafood is an excellent option for those who don't like poultry or red meat. It contains a lot of protein but is low in fat and calories, and it contains many different vitamins and minerals. When purchasing seafood, it's recommended to buy fresh fish from a good source – preferably someone who has a high volume of customers, so you know the fish hasn't been sitting in the display case more than 2 days. If the fish smells terrible, it will taste bad too, so don't buy it. And skip any cooked fish displayed next to raw fish to avoid cross-contamination. If you can't find fresh fish, your next best option is frozen. Just make sure that you cook it right away after defrosting it.

## Condiments

**Yogurt**: It may surprise you to hear that yogurt can be a condiment, but it's frequently used that way in this eating plan, where a small scoop can be a topping. It can also be incorporated into sauces and poured over some dishes. You'll find that some recipes you encounter in your new Mediterranean style of eating require the richer flavor of whole-milk yogurt, but you can use low-fat or nonfat yogurt in some dishes. Greek yogurt, which is thicker and creamier than regular yogurt, is typical in Mediterranean countries – and around the world. It contains live and active bacteria that aid your digestive and immune systems. Greek yogurt can be an ingredient or a side dish to many breakfast, lunch or dinner recipes. This type of yogurt, in particular, is perfect for making thick and creamy Tzatziki sauce, which can be used as a dip or sauce for dishes like kebobs, gyros, and falafel.

**Tahini:** This paste is made from ground sesame seeds. It can be included as a topping by itself or incorporated into certain sauces and dips, like hummus and baba ghanoush.

**Pomegranate molasses:** This thick, syrupy condiment, made by simply reducing pomegranate juice, is used to add tang to many dishes. If you cannot find it in a store, it is easy enough to learn to make it on your own.

**Preserved lemons:** This little-known ingredient comes from North Africa. It is very easy to make preserved lemons, but they take several weeks to cure. Once cured, you can keep them for up to six months in the refrigerator without worrying about them spoiling. However, if necessary, you can make a quick substitute: Combine four 2-inch strips of lemon zest, minced, 1 teaspoon of lemon juice, ½ teaspoon of water, ¼ teaspoon of sugar, and ¼ teaspoon of salt. Microwave this mixture at 50 percent power until the liquid evaporates, about 1 ½ minute, stirring and mashing the lemon with the back of a spoon every 30 seconds. This method makes about 1 tablespoon of a preserved lemon substitute.

**Dukkah:** This condiment stems from Egypt. It consists of a combination of spices, seeds, and nuts, and it can be used to add a distinctive flavor to many dishes. It can also be simply added to olive oil to be used as a dip for bread. Not all forms of dukkah are the same. As you become more comfortable with preparing Mediterranean cuisine, you may find that you prefer to make your own dukkah.

**Honey:** Honey is a natural sweetener that's superb for use in baked goods, desserts, breakfast, teas, and coffee. It contains 70 to 80 percent monosaccharides, fructose, and glucose, which give it its sweet flavor. Research has shown that the antiseptic and antibacterial properties of honey can help with a cold or heal wounds.

**Waters:** Have you ever had orange blossom water or rose water? Neither has a substantial nutritional value, but they both have intense flavors and add an exotic flavor element to any dessert or drink. You can find them at specialty food stores. They're fairly inexpensive.

**Syrups:** Syrups in Mediterranean cooking are most commonly used for desserts, as a topping. Simple syrup, for example, is made from simmering sugar, water, a bit of lemon juice, and a flavoring such as orange blossom water or rose water. Then you can drizzle it on phyllo pastries, fruit, or yogurt to sweeten.

## All About Olive Oil

Perhaps the most significant ingredient of Mediterranean cuisine is olive oil. Only produced from crushed and pressed olives, there may be no other food product that is quite so distinctive to this eating plan than this one. Olive oil is classified according to grades that indicate its quality. The highest quality is called "extra-virgin," and this is the type that should be used for all of your cooking and raw applications of olive oil in this eating plan. Its flavors vary wildly depending on which olives were used for producing it and how ripe they were at harvest time. It is made in several parts of the Mediterranean; however, California is also a top producer of olive oil in North America.

You may remember that olive oil helps support the goal of incorporating more healthy unsaturated fats into your diet. The use of this fat instead of butter or margarine is far healthier for your heart. Additionally, since it is a food derived from a plant, it contains antioxidants and other essential nutrients that help your body fight diseases like cancer and diabetes.

Extra-virgin olive oil is known as an important component of dressings and a tasty dip for pieces of bread. On top of those well-known uses, it is also often drizzled over vegetables and pasta, incorporated into sauces for meats and fish, and used for cooking ingredients of soups and stews. For a heart-healthy application in desserts, try replacing butter with olive oil in pastries. For example, a pie or tart crust made from olive oil can have a surprisingly savory flavor and tender texture.

## Buying and Storing Olive Oil

Finding the right extra-virgin olive oil for your cooking purposes can be confusing. Unfortunately, standards for olive oil quality are typically voluntary and rarely enforced, so the bottles labeled "extra virgin" may be a company's lower-quality olive oil that is being passed off at a higher price than it deserves.

Extra virgin olive oils range wildly in price, color, and quality, so it's hard to know which to buy. While many things can affect the style and flavor of olive oil, the main factors are the variety of olive and the time of harvest (earlier means greener, more bitter, and pungent); weather and processing also play a part. The best-quality olive oil comes from olives pressed as quickly as possible without heat. The use of heat in pressing the olives coaxes more oil from the olives, but it sacrifices the excellent taste of the product.

Since there is a vast number of different types of extra virgin olive oils for sale on grocery store shelves, some of the experts at America's Test Kitchen took it upon themselves to try and narrow down the options for confused consumers. They came up with a plan to find the best "everyday" extra virgin olive oil and the best "high-end" product so they could confidently recommend specific products.

To find the best "everyday" olive oil, the test participants tasted 10 lower-priced olive oils in various applications. The testers also sent each of the oils to a lab to be evaluated for quality and accuracy of grading. Finally, they had 10 highly-trained olive oil tasters for their opinion on each variety.

Ultimately, one oil was the clear winner over the other "supermarket" brands: California Olive Ranch Everyday Extra Virgin Olive Oil. They discovered that this product's superiority could be attributed to this company's vigilance and control over quality and speed in every step of production. Since olives change flavors rapidly after they are picked, speed is highly relevant in getting from picking the olives to pressing them into oil, then quickly bottling the oil before it oxidizes and spoils. At $9.99 for a 500 mL bottle, it is more expensive than some inferior oils found in the grocery store, but it is much more economical than the high-end oils.

It may surprise you to discover that the most expensive high-end oils are not always the best ones. The high-end oil that came out on top for America's Test Kitchen is called Gaea Fresh. This oil was produced in Greece, and at $18.99 for a 500 mL bottle, is surprisingly affordable when compared with other "high-end" olive oils. Tasters were impressed by this oil's flavor, which was strong but well-balanced. It is recommended that you use this high-end oil in raw applications only, where strong flavor counts.

Of course, you're bound to find countless other opinions about which is the best olive oil for your cooking needs. As you grow more experienced in using and tasting olive oil, you may even come up with your favorite brand of extra virgin olive oil. Feel free to experiment and research to your heart's content!

## Keeping Your Olive Oil Fresh

Three criteria will help you decide on the quality of your extra-virgin olive oil before purchasing it and help you keep it as fresh as possible.

**Oil Origin:** Bottlers, often print where their oil has been sourced from on the label; look for oil that has been sourced from a single country.

**Harvest Date:** Even though some oils may have a "best if used by" date, the harvest date is a more accurate descriptor of its freshness. Typically, olive oil starts to degrade about a year and a half after the olives were harvested. You'll want to buy a bottle that has the most recent date, and certainly one within the last year. If there is no harvest date, it may not be a good idea to buy that bottle at all. Since olives are harvested during the fall and winter in the Northern Hemisphere, you may only be able to find bottles that list the previous year.

**Dark Glass:** Only dark glass adequately shields the oil from damage caused by light and air. Clear glass and clear plastic just do not have what it takes to keep your olive oil as fresh and pristine as possible.

## To Store

You should never keep your olive oil out where it will be exposed to light. Since it is a plant product, it contains chlorophyll, which will oxidize in sunlight. Additionally, make sure not to keep your olive oil where it will be exposed to unnecessary heat, such as a cabinet right next to the oven. It is best kept in a cool, dark cabinet, but not in the refrigerator, where it will become cloudy and thick. Once you open a bottle of olive oil, you need to use it within three months, but an unopened bottle can be kept for up to a year.

You only need your sense of smell to check your olive oil for its freshness. Pour a little of it out and smell it. The smell of rancid olive oil tends to remind people of either stale walnuts or crayons. If this is the smell that greets you, it's time to throw the bottle out.

Now that you've learned how to begin making the necessary changes for embarking on this new phase in your life, it's time to look specifically at how the Mediterranean diet can help you in your weight loss goals if that is your desire.

# Chapter 5: The Mediterranean Diet and Weight Loss

The Mediterranean diet – a well-balanced diet that includes healthy fats and complex carbohydrates – offers the best alternative to popular fad diets if you're looking to lose weight without sacrificing your health. By pairing this eating plan with lower stress and increased exercise, you can do more than just lose a few pounds; you can also reduce your blood pressure, cholesterol, and blood sugar. As you've already read in earlier chapters of this book, those are just the beginning of the benefits.

One of the essential influence's diets can have upon health is by merely establishing weight control. Being overweight can damage every system in the body and is a risk factor for all our most serious, debilitating diseases. The Mediterranean diet helps one maintain a healthy weight by providing complex carbohydrates, fiber, and protein to help you feel full and to slow digestion, so you feel satisfied for longer.

People who live in the Mediterranean region *and* follow a Mediterranean diet and lifestyle, are leaner than their American counterparts for the following reasons:

- Exercise is a part of their everyday lives.
- They consume foods with high fiber content, like fruits, vegetables, beans, nuts, and whole grains. These foods lead to high satiety, the feeling of being full.
- They avoid trans fats, which are associated with weight gain and obesity. Instead, they eat healthy fats, like monounsaturated fat and omega-3 fat. Fat consumption, in the form of olive oil, nuts, and fish, also leads to satiety.

- They consume complex carbohydrates rather than simple carbohydrates, and they avoid refined sugars, which are linked with obesity. Complex carbohydrates also help the consumer feel full longer.
- Food is not "super-sized" in Mediterranean countries like it is in America. It is the quality of food, not the quantity of food, that makes a good meal!

## Calories and Weight Loss

The secret to weight loss is simple: burn more calories than you consume. Quite simply, Americans consume too many calories! We eat large meals and then a snack in the evening while we sit and watch TV. This excessive caloric intake combined with our sedentary lifestyle is the reason that obesity is a significant public health threat. Although the Mediterranean diet is not one that is geared towards obsessive calorie-counting, there are several tips you can follow that will help you reduce your overall calorie intake, without having to write down every calorie you put in your mouth.

### Portion Control

We must learn to eat smart. First, we need to limit the portions of the food we eat. Over the years, restaurant portions and packaged food portions have gradually increased in size. The average bagel now weighs four to five ounces (equal to four or five slices of bread), cookies are the size of saucers, and an order of pasta in a restaurant would once have fed a family of four. To determine what an "average" serving of packaged food should really be, check the nutrition label. You may be surprised to learn that the "single" packaged food portion you've been assuming was for one is actually intended for two – or more. You don't need to weigh or measure foods, but use common sense, and learn to eyeball right portions. For instance, a medium orange is about the size of a tennis ball, and a three-ounce piece of meat is about the size of the palm of your hand.

In Chapter 2, you read the recommended serving sizes and number of servings in each of the Mediterranean diet's food groups. As suggested in that chapter, you can use your body size, activity level, and weight loss goals as guides to the number of servings you should have within the guidelines. If you stick to these recommendations, you may be able to lose weight without counting a single calorie. However, if you have trouble losing weight by merely controlling portions and number of servings, you can learn more about counting calories later in this chapter.

## Increased Physical Activity

Besides learning to limit our portions, we also need to start exercising. In chapter 4 you read several tips on slowly incorporating more physical activity into your life. If you struggle with motivation, try to remind yourself that you are doing this for more than just your waistline – it's essential to exercise if you wish to live as long and as healthy of a life as possible. By starting and maintaining a habit of daily exercise, you'll help ensure that you'll be around to enjoy life with your family and friends for as long as possible.

Another tip for increasing your motivation to exercise is to find someone who will help you remain accountable. Finding a workout buddy not only helps you when you struggle to get off the couch and get active, but it also adds elements of fun and social interaction to your exercise routine.

## More Whole Foods, Fewer Processed Foods

Finally, we must also replace processed food, refined sugar, trans fats, and saturated fats with healthier, lower-calorie whole foods – as in the Mediterranean diet. Also, because the concentration is on fresh food, you're not eating commercially-made products that are higher in calories as well as designed to compel you to overeat and create irresistible cravings. It's also easy to follow because it doesn't involve an extreme diet makeover, and – as you'll see when you start trying recipes – it tastes so good!

## Counting Calories

As previously stated, the Mediterranean diet is not one that necessarily lends itself to obsessive calorie counting. Ideally, you'll find that by focusing on eating fresh and whole foods, limiting portion size, avoiding processed foods, and increasing your activity level, you will begin to lose weight naturally. However, if you find that the scale won't budge, or you reach a "plateau" in your weight loss – a point at which your weight loss stalls and you can't lose that last 10, 20, or 30 pounds – it may become necessary to begin counting calories, at least until you become accustomed to estimating your body's nutritional needs.

### Determining Your Metabolic Needs

The first step towards learning how many calories you should be consuming to lose weight, is to figure out your basal metabolic rate, or BMR. This amount of energy (in calories) that you would burn if you were sleeping all day long. Below are the steps for figuring out this equation:

1.  Determine your weight in centimeters. You can either measure it in centimeters or, if you know how tall you are in inches, multiply this number by 2.54. For example, if you are 63 in. in height, multiply that by 2.54, and the answer is approximately 160 cm.

2.  Determine your weight in kilograms. You can get your weight in pounds and convert it to kg by dividing it by 2.2. For a 135-pound person, you would divide 135 by 2.2 for an answer of about 61.4 kg.

3. If you are a male, use this equation to get your BMR in calories per day:

> BMR = (cm of height multiplied by 6.25) + (kg of weight multiplied by 9.99) − (your age multiplied by 4.92) + 5.
> With the above numbers, if you are 36 years old, the equation would look like this:
> BMR = (160 x 6.25) + (61.4 x 9.99) − (36 x 4.92) + 5 = 1000 + 613.39 − 177.12 + 5 = 1441.27 calories per day

4. If you are a female, use this equation to get your BMR in calories per day:

> BMR = (cm of height multiplied by 6.25) + (kg of weight multiplied by 9.99) − (your age multiplied by 4.92) − 161
> With the above numbers, if you are 36 years old, the equation would look like this:
> BMR = (160 x 6.25) + (61.4 x 9.99) − (36 x 4.92) − 161 = 1000 + 613.39 − 177.12 − 161 = 1275.27 calories per day

Next, you need to use your BMR and daily activity level to determine your total energy expenditure (TEE) per day or the amount of energy (in calories) your body burns each day at your current activity level. The BMR result is multiplied by a factor that is used to estimate your physical activity level (PAL) to determine their TEE, as follows:

- If your lifestyle is sedentary or includes only very light activity, such as working in an office, multiply your BMR by 1.53.
- If your lifestyle is active or moderately active, such as standing work in a factory, housecleaning, or if you get a

moderate amount of daily exercise, multiply your BMR by 1.76.

- If your lifestyle is vigorously active, with extremely strenuous physical labor or intense and lengthy daily exercise, multiply your BMR by 2.25.

For example, for the woman with the BMR of 1275.27 calories per day above, let's say she has a moderately active job. She would multiply 1275.27 by 1.76 to get approximately 2,244 calories. This is the approximate amount that this woman needs to eat each day if she wishes to maintain her current weight of 135 pounds.

## Determining Your Weight Loss Needs

If you are trying to lose weight, the only way to do it is by consuming fewer calories than you burn. There are two ways to do this – either you can incorporate more vigorous physical activity into your daily life and keep eating the same number of calories, or you can decrease the amount of calories you eat per day. You can choose to do both, but you must be vigilant to make sure you aren't making too many drastic changes. If you end up in a situation in which you are consuming drastically too few calories for your body's needs, you can end up with serious health complications. At the very least, your body might go into "starvation mode," in which it conserves every precious ounce of energy in a desperate attempt to stay alive. In this case, you may not end up losing as much weight as you had hoped. The key is to strike a balance, in which you have enough of a calorie deficit to lose weight, while still consuming enough energy to fuel your body adequately.

The safest way to determine how many calories to cut is by using math once again. A wise and safe strategy in weight loss is to try and lose 1 to 2 pounds per week. The loss of one pound requires a deficit of 3,500 calories. Spread out over a week, and that makes a deficit of 500 calories per day. You could either try to exercise enough to about 500 calories of extra energy each day, eat about 500 fewer calories daily, or strike a balance by cutting 250 calories and burning an extra 250 calories.

For example, with the same example woman who weighs 135 pounds and needs to eat 2,244 calories each day to maintain this weight. Let's say she wishes to lose about one pound per week until she reaches her goal weight of 120 pounds. To accomplish this, she has three options:

1. She could maintain the same activity level and eat 1,744 calories each day for a daily calorie deficit of 500.
2. She could find a daily activity that burns an extra 500 calories each day, while still consuming 2, 244 calories each day.
3. She could eat 1,996 calories each day and find an activity that burns an extra 250 calories each day.

With any of the three above options, the woman ends up with a weekly reduction that totals 3,500 calories, which should lead to a weight loss of about a pound each week.

## Help with Counting Calories

Each recipe in this book reports an accurate calorie count per serving, along with protein, carbohydrates, and fat content. There are only 20 recipes to get you started here, but you can find an infinite number of Mediterranean diet recipes on the internet and in other books once you are ready to start trying more dishes. Many of these recipes will also include calorie counts.

If you want to try a recipe that does not report calories, use common sense and compare it to other similar recipes. Or you can get incredibly detailed and calculate the calories of the entire recipe by adding all the ingredients together and dividing the total by the number of servings.

There are a lot of phone and tablet apps that will help you keep track of your calories and encourage you when you meet your goals each day. You can also do internet searches on calorie counts for different foods and meals, and you will often find remarkably accurate results.

## If the Scale Still Won't Budge – Troubleshooting

In some cases, you may feel like you are doing everything right and *still* not losing weight. Or perhaps you started off with rapid weight loss, and now you have reached the dreaded plateau. If this becomes the situation for you, you can try a few different strategies:

- Consult your doctor. He may want to run blood tests to rule out any underlying metabolic issues.
- Change up your exercise routine. As the body gets used to any particular form of activity, it becomes more and more efficient at accomplishing the same goals. This means that it gradually burns fewer calories. If you change your exercise routine, you "confuse" your muscles, leading them to work harder and burn more energy again.
- Drink more water. Your body is better at metabolizing energy if it is well hydrated. Just in case you needed one more reason to stay hydrated, there you have it!
- Eat just a little less. Try cutting out one snack, one dessert, or half of a side dish per day to see if just a little more of a deficit helps. Again, you should not take your calorie deficit to extremes!
- Eat just a little more. It is possible your body is too deprived and is beginning to enter into the aforementioned "starvation mode." Many people have discovered that, by eating 200 or so additional healthy

calories (lean protein, vegetables, fruit, or whole grains) each day, they were able to meet their weight loss goals.

- Just focus on enjoying your life, healthy nutrition, and surrounding yourself with family and friends. Many people have found that, when they focus on enjoying the positive things of life and stop obsessively counting calories, they can lose weight without much effort gradually.

If you still find yourself plagued by troublesome weight and nothing is working, it may be time to return to your doctor or consult a registered dietician (RD). These professionals can give you the expert guidance you need to troubleshoot your diet and get you pointed in the right direction.

## Eating Out on This Diet

Sometimes eating out can be a problem no matter what diet plan or lifestyle you're following. Most items on restaurant menus are filled with salt, fat, and preservatives, making them off-limits.

However, you can still dine out on the Mediterranean diet. Find places to eat that align with your healthy eating habits, such as fresh fruit and vegetable items instead of fried or sauce-laden sides. Also, choose menu items that aren't cooked in butter or heavy sauces, and ask for sauces or dressing to be served on the side so you can control how much you consume.

Many restaurants print the calorie content of their dishes on the menu now, making it easier for us to make health-conscious decisions. If nutritional information is not available on a menu, most chain restaurants have this information listed on their websites. Having this information ahead of time can help you make a smart decision before you even get to the restaurant.

That way, you are less likely to fall prey to tempting choices or advertised specials when you arrive at the restaurant.

Ask your server for recommendations, too, or see if he or she could ask the chef to make adjustments for you. You could request a lighter dressing or ask for something to be grilled instead of fried. Remember, you're paying for it, so don't be afraid to ask for what you want politely.

# Chapter 6: In Case You're Considering Other Diet

In America, we are often enticed by "quick fix" diets that promise rapid, sustained weight loss. The problem with most of these diets, is that they have no scientific basis, nor is there any long-term data demonstrating their effectiveness regarding steady weight loss or long-term health. Many of these diets can be defined as fad diets, most of which promise that you'll see easy, sudden weight loss. The sad truth is that although some of them may result in initial weight loss, the weight is often quickly gained back. The initial weight loss may not even be healthy weight loss, either. Starving yourself can also lead to weight loss, but it deprives you of the vitamins and nutrients you need to live and can cause permanent damage to your body.

Throughout time, waves of dietary change have come and gone low-fat, nonfat, low-carb, high-carb, vegan, Paleo, etc. These diets are marketed with the promise to promote health and happiness, but they are usually entrenched with all-or-nothing claims, gimmicks, and short-lived dietary plans that are not enjoyable or sustainable. They simply don't (and can't) last.

The Mediterranean diet works. It's easy, and there's no deprivation of any food group. There are recommended *restrictions* of certain foods that aren't beneficial to health, but there are ample choices to maintain variety and satiety for all palettes. Research consistently proves that eating a heart-healthy Mediterranean diet will slash cancer and stroke risks, eradicate preventable diets, and boost the quality of life – not just your quantity of years.

It's no surprise that when following a Mediterranean diet, which promotes healthy fats, produce, whole grains, and seafood, you have lower risks of heart disease and cholesterol, have lower body mass indexes, and experience more heart-healthy benefits. By sticking to healthy portions of fresh food in its natural state, you will obtain all the nutrients needed to nourish the body.

But how can a diet rich in health be healthier than what average Americans eat? Because those fats don't come from animals. Americans consume *saturated* fat, which hinders health. Saturated fats raise cholesterol and can contribute to heart disease. People of the Mediterranean eat *monounsaturated* fat from plant sources, which promotes heart health. Monounsaturated fats help lower levels of cholesterol and reduce our risk of heart disease and stroke. In the famous Seven Countries Study, Ancel Keys observed that the people of Crete, Greece consumed as much as a ½ cup of olive oil per day, per person! He also observed that heart disease rates in the Mediterranean regions of Italy, Spain, and France were incredibly low. It's not always about calories, fat, or protein. It's about the *source* of your food and the *quality* of our ingredients.

Despite the substantial scientific evidence behind the Mediterranean diet, you still may be fascinated by one of the many popular diets that have been publicized and popularized in recent years. Here, we'll take a look at some of those diets and discover how the Mediterranean diet stacks up against each one. In some cases, you may be able to find a healthy compromise that combines the Mediterranean diet with another eating plan. In other cases, the Mediterranean way of eating comes out as the clear winner.

## The Ketogenic Diet

This is a more trendy diet, recently popularized by social media users, consists of a high-fat, low-carbohydrate, medium-protein eating plan. After you have restricted your consumption of carbohydrates to minimal levels, your metabolism will shift to a process called ketosis, in which your body mobilizes its own carbohydrate stores for fuel because it is not getting enough energy from carbohydrates. The result of this process is thought to be increased burning of the body's fat stores.

With this food pattern, you aim to consume approximately 75% of your calories from fats like avocado, butter, oils, and bacon. Your consumption of fats is almost unlimited, so you get to enjoy some fat-rich choices that most other diets would never allow. You eat about 15 to 20 percent of your calories in protein, which is a moderate amount. Carbohydrate intake is severely limited to only 5 to 10 percent of your diet. This is approximately equivalent to the level of carbohydrates you can find in a couple of apples each day.

By comparison, on the Mediterranean diet, about 50 to 60 percent of your intake is healthy carbohydrates that can be found in fruits, vegetables, and whole grain sources. Fat makes up about a 25 to 35 percent of the diet, with an emphasis on consuming heart-healthy unsaturated fats, found in olive oil, fish, and nuts. Saturated fats, found mainly in animal products, are kept to a minimum.

As you have read throughout this book, the Mediterranean diet is backed by thousands of scientific studies and has been proven to reduce the risk of death from several very svere health issues. On the flip side, the ketogenic diet was initially developed as nutritional therapy for epileptic children! At the time, it was used to help manage seizures in these children. It was never designed for weight loss or the management of other health issues.

The Ketogenic diet is a more challenging and painful way of eating! It limits healthy carbohydrates like whole grains, fruits, and vegetables so severely that it can lead to dangerous deficiencies in essential nutrients. For the sake of your body's natural energy levels, it is challenging, if not impossible, to stick to a low-carb diet for a long time. Additionally, the high levels of saturated fat consumed in the ketogenic diet are dangerous for the health of your cardiovascular system. Eating a lot of animal products rich in saturated fats has been shown to increase your risk of health issues related to circulation and heart health.

Clearly, the winner in this comparison is the Mediterranean diet. It is a safe and healthy solution for long-term weight management and the best chances of enjoying a long, disease-free life. You may be able to lose weight more rapidly with the ketogenic diet, but it is not a wise choice for long-term health or establishing a pattern of wise nutritional decisions.

## The Paleo Diet

This diet, which follows the eating patterns of modern man's Stone Age ancestors, is relatively new. Enthusiasts of this diet claim that our bodies were not designed to digest much of what we eat today, and they promote cutting out whole food groups, including grains, dairy, legumes, added sugar, and added salt. The goals of the Paleo diet are the improvement of overall health, weight loss, and decreased risk of diseases.

The Paleo diet has a couple of things in common with the Mediterranean diet. First, both eating plans emphasize the consumption of fresh, whole foods instead of processed foods that contain excessive sugars, salt, and other unhealthy additives. Both diets include nuts, vegetables, fruits, and lean protein sources, all of which have benefits to maintaining a healthy weight, heart health, and lowering the risk of diseases like type 2 diabetes.

However, by cutting out entire food groups, the Paleo diet comes with some risk factors that should be taken into account. Because it excludes dairy, people who follow this diet risk calcium deficiencies. Calcium can be found in leafy greens, but the highest concentration of this critical mineral is in dairy products. Most typical Americans cannot consume the quantity of dark leafy greens required to get their daily recommended amount of calcium. Without enough calcium, we risk developing osteoporosis, numbness in our fingers and toes, convulsions, muscle cramps, and abnormal heart rhythm.

The Paleo diet also cuts out grains and legumes, both of which play essential roles in the Mediterranean diet. Both food groups have been shown to aid digestion, contain vital nutrients, and help prevent serious diseases. Additionally, the Paleo diet can be too high in protein for the average person, which can affect your kidney function.

The bottom line is that the Paleo diet, although not as dangerous as the ketogenic diet, does not stand up to the Mediterranean diet as a well-established and balanced way of eating for long-term health. Additionally, we must consider the fact that significant evolution has taken place in the human digestive system since the Stone Age. Perhaps our ancestors could not have digested grains, legumes, and dairy products. However, now those food groups, in healthy amounts, are easily absorbed by most people and supply important sources of vital nutrients.

## Low-Carbohydrate Diets

Both the ketogenic and Paleo diets are forms of low-carbohydrate diets, with the ketogenic diet being a much more extreme version of low-carb eating. Another low-carb diet is the Atkins Diet, which was first publicized more than 30 years ago. This somewhat old fad diet is remarkably similar to the ketogenic diet in that it allows and even encourages the consumption of foods that are high in saturated fat and protein.

There is no need to spend much time comparing the Mediterranean diet with the Atkins or other low-carb diets because the basics have already been covered in the last two sections. Depriving the body of essential nutrients found in fruits, vegetables, and whole grains can ultimately be detrimental to health. Replacing carbohydrates with too much fat (especially saturated fat) and protein puts a strain on the kidneys and heart. The Atkins diet and other low-carbohydrate diets may lead to initial rapid weight loss, but studies and anecdotal evidence has shown that this weight loss often slows and sometimes reverses.

## Intermittent Fasting

This recent health trend, in contrast with other diets, does not specify what foods to eat and avoid. Instead, it dictates eating patterns in which periods of fasting are alternated with periods of eating.

There are a few patterns of intermittent fasting that are currently popular, and those who wish to try this strategy should take their health, metabolism, gender, activity level, and other lifestyle factors into account when deciding which eating pattern to follow. One pattern is called the 5:2 pattern, in which the dieter normally eats during five days of the week, and drastically restricts his calorie intake for 2 non-consecutive days of each week. Another pattern, the 16/8 method, involves fasting for 16 hours each day and eating normally for only 8 hours a day. A third method is called "eat-stop-eat," and involves fasting for a full 24 hours at a time, once or twice a week.

Intermittent fasting has been shown to help stimulate weight loss because of changes in metabolism and hormone levels that take place when a person enters a fasting phase. Additionally, because all these methods result in the overall reduction of calorie intake, the dieter should lose weight, as long as he does not compensate by eating excessive amounts of food during the "normal eating" periods. Many people find this method easier than other diets because it does not deem any food groups "off-limits." As a result, intermittent fasting can be highly successful in helping you achieve lasting weight loss.

If you do not have any significant health concerns in which fasting causes problems, there is no reason that you should not consider combining the Mediterranean diet with intermittent fasting. Be sure to consult your doctor before embarking on this method, though. He may recommend testing or have some advice about the best fasting and eating pattern for you to follow.

Additionally, if you follow the Mediterranean diet during your eating periods, you will be helping to ensure that your body receives the best nutrition possible during the meals that you do consume. Getting adequate healthy nutrition will help set you up for success in this method, because your body will have received enough fuel to help you make it through the fasting periods.

## The DASH and MIND Diets

The DASH, or "Dietary Attempts to Stop Hypertension," diet was initially publicized to help hypertensive patients lower their blood pressure. The Mediterranean diet and the DASH diets have ranked extremely high in recent years as the best eating plans to follow for long-term health.

The two diets are very similar to each other, too. They both encourage the consumption of healthy fats, lean protein sources, whole grains, nuts, legumes, fruits, and vegetables. The critical difference seems to be that the DASH diet allows for more low-fat dairy than the Mediterranean diet.

If you're interested in pursuing both the Mediterranean diet and the DASH diet, there is an easy solution for you. The MIND diet, which is an acronym for the "Mediterranean-DASH Intervention for Neurodegenerative Delay," is a hybrid of these two highly effective diets that aims to reduce the risks of dementia and age-related declines in brain health. The premise behind this diet is that both the Mediterranean and DASH diets have been proven to lower blood pressure, and reduce the risk of several life-threatening diseases. However, neither was created with the goal of improving brain function and preventing dementia. By taking the most brain-healthy elements of both diets, the experts believe they have crafted the best diet for preventing neurodegenerative diseases. The foods recommended on the MIND diet are backed by countless studies and research reviews that show their benefits to brain health.

Rather than focusing on calories or other restrictions, the MIND diet emphasizes the consumption of certain foods over others. Specifically, it recommends that participants eat a lot of green, leafy vegetables along with other vegetables, wine (in moderation, olive oil, fish, berries, poultry, whole grains, and nuts. There are recommended daily, or weekly serving amounts for each of these foods. This diet recommends avoiding butter and margarine, cheese, red meat, fried food, and processed junk food and sweets.

Since the MIND, DASH, and Mediterranean diets are so remarkably similar, you should feel free to try any of the three, depending on your health goals. If you just want a healthy eating plan that helps you enjoy life and reduce your overall risk of disease, the Mediterranean diet is for you. If you have concerns about high blood pressure, you may want to learn more about the DASH diet. If you are focused on protecting your brain health, you should think about following the MIND diet.

The bottom line of this chapter is that it's hard to beat the Mediterranean diet when it comes to an eating plan that promotes long-term health and the enjoyment of life without restricting entire food groups. However, there are variations of this diet that were crafted for people with specific health concerns. If you are one of those people, you can still enjoy the Mediterranean way of life while focusing on your own particular needs.

# Chapter 7: Easy Mediterranean Recipes

*NOTE: At the end of each recipe, you'll find a low-carbohydrate variation and a low-sodium variation.

## Breakfast Selections

### Savory Breakfast Salad

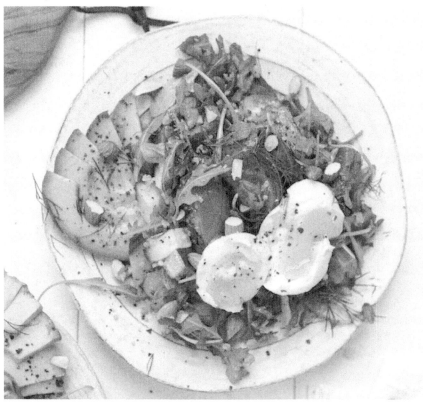

Total Prep and Cooking Time: 15-20 minutes

### Nutrition (per serving)
Calories: 519
Fat: 39.4 g.
Carbohydrates: 29.1 g.
Protein: 19.1 g.

Serves 4 people

Although eating a salad for breakfast may seem like a strange idea, so does eating cold leftover pizza from last night – and yet, many of us have woken up on a Saturday morning and eaten a cold slice straight from the fridge. So why not try a healthy option and go for a salad? This dish is loaded with tasty breakfast bites like soft-boiled eggs, tomato, and avocado. Peppery arugula is a delicious non-bread option for soaking up the runny yolks. The healthy fat from avocado and olive oil will help you feel full and energetic until lunch time. To top it off, crunchy almonds and fiber-laden quinoa add even more protein and flavor! Salad for breakfast? Yes, please!

## Component
4 eggs, large
2 c. cherry tomatoes, cut in half; or chopped heirloom or Roma tomatoes
10 c. arugula rinsed and patted dry
½ of a seedless cucumber, roughly chopped
1 c. cooked and cooled quinoa
1 c. almonds, chopped (optional: toast the almonds for a flavor boost)
1 large avocado, sliced
½ c. mixed green herbs (examples: mint, dill, or basil)
1 lemon
Salt and pepper
2 Tbsp. extra-virgin olive oil, for drizzling

## Preparation:
1.  Soft-boil the eggs. Heat a pot of cold water until it boils, then lower the heat until the liquid is simmering (gently bubbling, or just below boiling). Then gently place the eggs in the water with a large spoon and leave them in

the simmering water for 6 minutes. Remove them promptly from the pot and run them under cold water immediately. Set the eggs aside; peel them when you are ready to use them.

2. Place the following ingredients in a large bowl: chopped tomatoes, chopped cucumber, cold cooked quinoa, and arugula. Toss to combine, then drizzle about half of the oil over it. Season with the ground pepper and salt, then toss again.

3. Divide the mixture from the bowl between four plates. Next, peel the eggs and cut them in half. Soon after, top each salad with one-halved egg and ¼ of the sliced avocado. Sprinkle the mixed herbs and almonds evenly over the top of the four salads. Top each salad by gently squeezing a little lemon juice over it, sprinkling a bit more salt and pepper (to taste), and drizzling the rest of the olive oil over it. Share and enjoy!

_Low-Carbohydrate Variation_: Cut the number of vegetables in half and eliminate the quinoa. Add one more egg per person and double the almonds.

_Low-Sodium Variation:_ Do not use any salt.

# Almond-Honey Ricotta and Peaches on English Muffin

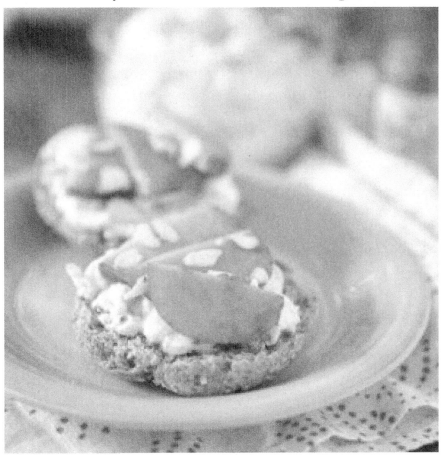

Total Prep and Cooking Time: 10 minutes

## Nutrition (per serving)
Calories: 391
Fat: 17.4 g.
Carbohydrates: 46.8 g.
Protein: 16.6 g.

Serves 4 people

In contrast to some more savory breakfast dishes, this dish will satisfy anyone who wakes up with a craving for something sweet. The almonds and whole-wheat muffin, in addition to the fat from ricotta cheese, help give you sustainable energy. Peaches and honey add healthy sources of sweetness and vital nutrients to the start of your day. If you like to begin with a stack of syrupy pancakes, try this meal out for a healthy Mediterranean substitute.

## Components

4 whole-grain English muffins
1 c. whole milk ricotta
5 tsp honey
¼ tsp almond extract
½ c. sliced almonds
2 medium ripe peaches, pitted and sliced
orange zest (optional)

## Preparation

1. Separate the halves of the English muffins and toast them.
2. While the muffins are toasting, combine the following items in a small bowl: Ricotta cheese, 1 tsp. of the honey, almonds (set aside a few for sprinkling over the tops, if you like), almond extract, and orange zest (almonds). Stir it all together gently.
3. Spread approximately 1/8 of the mixture over each muffin half. Top with the peach slices, extra almonds that you set aside, and about ½ tsp. of honey per muffin half. Share and enjoy!

*Low-Carbohydrate Variation:* Serve the spread wrapped in a low-carb wrap. Use one peach instead of two. Add more almonds for increased satiety.

# Avocado, Smoked Salmon, and Poached Eggs on Toast

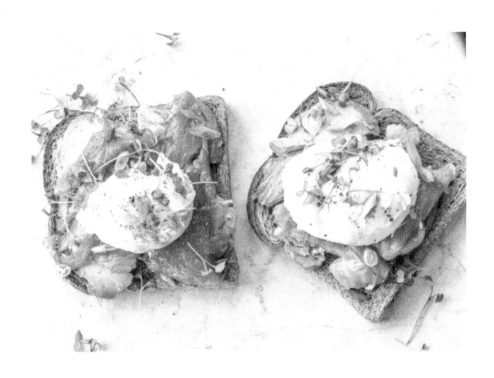

Total Prep and Cooking Time: 15-20 minutes

## **Nutrition (per serving)**
Calories: 463
Fat: 22.4 g.
Carbohydrates: 30.2 g.
Protein: 35.0 g.

Serves 1 person

When it comes to protein-packed breakfasts, this one carries the motherlode! Thanks to savory smoked salmon and two eggs, you'll definitely be satisfied by this tasty beginning to your day.

Add the creamy deliciousness of avocado and sharp peppery arugula, and your taste buds will be in heaven. While the smoked salmon is slightly less budget-friendly than most of the ingredients in this book, it is well worth the occasional splurge. This dish has everything you need for a satisfying start to a productive weekday, or a weekend brunch so tasty you can scarcely believe it's good for you.

## Components

2 slices whole grain bread, toasted
¼ large avocado
lemon juice, just a few drops
2 large eggs
¼ c. arugula
3 oz. smoked salmon
salt and pepper, if desired

## Preparation

1. Within a small bowl, mash up ¼ avocado thoroughly. Add the lemon juice, a tiny sprinkle of salt, stir and set this dish aside.
2. Poach the eggs, one at a time. See the instructions below if you've never poached an egg.
3. Divide the avocado mash in half and spread it over both slices of bread. Adorn the mashed avocado with the arugula leaves, then add ½ of the smoked salmon to each slice.
4. Gently place a poached egg on top of each slice, then sprinkle with salt and pepper to your liking.
5. Even though this meal is served on toast, you'll need a fork and knife to eat it!
6.

## Egg Poaching Directions:

1. Always poach eggs one at a time.

2. Heat a small pot of water until it is simmering (gently bubbling or almost boiling).
3. Crack the eggs cleanly into individual small bowls.
4. Use a large spoon to stir the simmering water until it moves smoothly in a circle, like a whirlpool.
5. Softly tip one egg into the swirling water and leave it in there for two minutes.
6. Remove the egg gently with a slotted spoon and put it in ice water for just about 10 seconds to stop the cooking process (this will keep the yolk runny).
7. Use a paper towel to pat the egg dry and use the edge of a spoon to cut off any wispy whites from around the egg.

*Low-Carbohydrate Variation:* Eliminate the bread and serve the other ingredients in a bowl. Double the avocado and consider adding more smoked salmon.

*Low-Sodium Variation:* Use fresh salmon that has been grilled, broiled, or poached instead of smoked salmon.

# Berry Good Greek Yogurt Pancakes

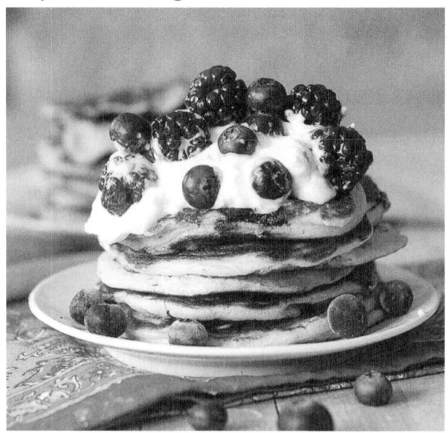

Total Prep and Cooking Time: 30 minutes

## Nutrition (per serving)
Calories: 301
Fat: 9.4 g.
Carbohydrates: 37.9 g.
Protein: 19.0 g.

Serves 6 people

Even though pancakes seem like a decadent treat that you shouldn't touch with a ten-foot pole when you're following a healthy eating plan, there actually is a way to enjoy them on the Mediterranean Diet! When you use whole wheat flour, limit the sugar, skip the syrup on top, and add protein-packed Greek yogurt to the mix, even pancakes can be relatively healthy! Topped with yummy berries, this family-friendly recipe is sure to be a crowd pleaser.

## Components

1 ¼ c. flour (preferably whole-wheat)

2 tsp. baking powder

1 tsp. of baking soda

¼ c. of sugar

¼ tsp. salt

3 c. nonfat plain Greek yogurt, divided in half

3 T. extra virgin olive oil

½ c. nonfat (skim) milk

1 ½ c. blueberries or other berries of your choosing

## Preparation

1. Within a mixing bowl, add all the following ingredients: flour, salt, and baking powder and soda. Combine them all together with a whisk.

2. Within a different bowl, add the oil, sugar, 1 ½ c. of the yogurt, and the milk. Use a whisk to blend them until smooth vigorously.

3. Gently combine the two mixtures (from step 1 and step 2) together. Use a spoon to form a smooth batter. For one option, gently stir in the berries. Otherwise, leave them out and use them for a topping when serving.

4. Warm a skillet or pancake griddle. Test by sprinkling water on the hot surface – if the water droplets sizzle on the surface, it's ready. Spray the hot surface with non-stick oil spray.

5. Pour the batter, ¼ c. at a time, onto the cooking surface. When bubbles on the wet surface pop and leave small holes, check the bottom edges to see if it's golden brown, then flip the pancake (use a wide spatula).

6. Place pancakes on a plate in a warm oven until ready to serve.

7. Serve topped with the remainder of the Greek yogurt and the berries (unless you incorporated them into the batter). Delicious!

*Low-Carbohydrate Variation*: The central part of this meal is carbohydrates, so you may want to avoid this dish altogether if you're cutting carbs. Instead, enjoy a bowl of Greek yogurt with a few blueberries.

*Low-Sodium Variation:* Eliminate the salt from the recipe.

**Veggie Egg Cups with Feta**

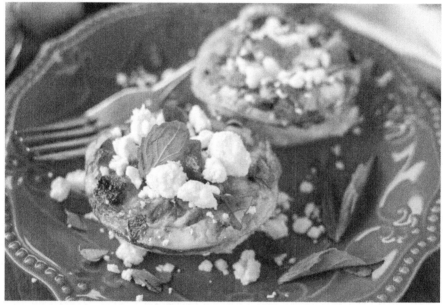

Total Prep and Cooking Time: 35-45 minutes

## Nutrition (per two egg cups)
Calories: 229
Fat: 17 grams
Carbohydrates: 4.6 grams
Protein: 15.3 grams

Serves 6 people

If you're a fan of preparing food a day or so before you need it, you'll love these delightful little egg cups! You can make them the night before and warm them up the next morning, or even serve them cold if you're in a hurry. The recipe serves six people, but we won't tell anyone if you eat it all yourself, spread out over six different mornings! If you're following a low-carb Mediterranean diet hybrid plan, this dish requires no modifications, as it barely contains any carbohydrates, to begin with. This version includes roasted red peppers and mushrooms, but you can feel free to substitute any other vegetable you have on hand.

## Components
10 large eggs
nonstick cooking spray
2/3 c. of nonfat (skim) milk
½ tsp. garlic powder
1/8 tsp. of salt
¼ tsp. ground pepper
1 ½ c. raw mushrooms, cleaned and chopped
1 ½ cup roasted red peppers, drained, rinsed, and dried
1 c. feta cheese
fresh basil leaves, for garnish

## Preparation
1. Warm up your oven until it reaches 350 degrees (F). You'll need a muffin tin with 12 cups that has been prepared with cooking spray.
2. Break all the eggs into a bowl, then add the milk, garlic powder, salt, and black pepper. Use a whisk to combine them all. Then add the mushrooms and peppers and stir until the vegetables are uniformly distributed.
3. Using a ladle, distribute the mixture evenly into the 12 cups of the muffin tin. It's okay if the cups are quite full.

4. Place muffin tin in the oven and leave for 25 minutes, or whenever the eggs look completely set (not runny or jiggly when the pan is shaken lightly).

5. Leave egg cups in the muffin tin to cool for 5 to 10 minutes. They will appear to deflate a little. Then remove them from the tin.

6. Serve 2 egg cups per serving. Top with feta cheese (divided into 6 portions) and basil leaves.

_Low-Carbohydrate Variation_: This is a low-carb recipe without any changes necessary.

_Low-Sodium Variation:_ Eliminate the salt in the recipe and sprinkle part-skim mozzarella on the egg cups instead of feta cheese.

# Lunch Selections

### Chickpea Lettuce Wraps

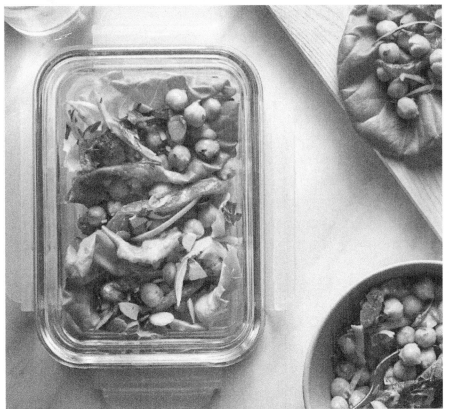

Total Prep and Cooking Time: 10 minutes

## <u>Nutrition (per serving)</u>
Calories: 516
Fat: 32.3 g.
Carbohydrates: 46.1 g.
Protein: 17.3 g.

Serves 4 people
This tasty lunch option easy to prepare ahead of time and bring to work, or you can make it at home for a light to share with family or friends. It's chock-full of the trademark Mediterranean flavors and nutrients, and it's guaranteed to satisfy. Although

it's high in carbohydrates, you must keep in mind that these are *healthy* carbohydrates, from vegetables and legumes. Your body will take its time breaking down the tasty, fiber-filled little chickpeas, and your taste buds will thank you for the flavor of the tangy tahini dressing and the crunch of toasted almonds in this no-cook, easy-to-prepare meal.

## Components

¼ c. tahini (a paste made from ground-up sesame seeds; refrigerate after opening)

¼ c. extra-virgin olive oil

1 teaspoon lemon zest

¼ c. juice from lemons (approximately the juice from 2 lemons)

1 ½ tsp. of pure maple syrup

¾ tsp. salt

½ teaspoon paprika

2 (15 oz.) cans chickpeas (no salt added), drained and rinsed

½ c. of Jarred sliced roasted red bell peppers, drained

½ c. thinly sliced shallots or green onions

12 large lettuce leaves – Bibb, butter, or Romaine are recommended, but any type that makes a good wrap will do

¼ c. chopped toasted almonds

2 Tbsp. parsley, fresh and minced

## Preparation

1. Place the sheet of meatballs on the middle rack of the heated oven and bake them 20-22 minutes. They should be golden brown before you take them out of the oven. Allow them to cool off outside the oven.

2. While the meatballs bake, make the yogurt dip. Add all the components of the sauce to a small bowl and whisk them together until thoroughly combined. Cover the bowl and chill until ready to serve.

3. Keep meatballs and yogurt in the refrigerator until ready to serve. The meatballs will keep for 3 to 4 days, and the dip will keep for 7 to 10 days.

4. Enjoy!

*Low-Carbohydrate Variation:* This is a low-carb recipe. You can use more lentils and fewer breadcrumbs if you like, but this may change the texture too much.

*Low-Sodium Variation:* Eliminate the table salt. Use mozzarella instead of feta cheese.

## Quinoa Chicken Power Bowl

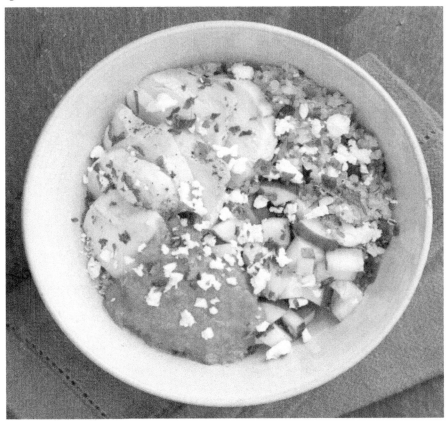

Total Prep and Cooking Time: 30 minutes

## Nutrition (per serving)

Calories: 520
Fat: 27 g.
Carbohydrates: 31 g.
Protein: 34 g.

Serves 4 people

Fresh ingredients seem to come together magically in this well-balanced, nutritious dish. This is another lunch that travels well and can be prepared in advance. Just cook the components ahead of time, bring them to work, and assemble the parts just before eating. You'll be wowed by how delicious a protein-packed power bowl can be when you taste the spices that blend easily into a delicious sauce.

## **Components**
1 pound of chicken breasts (boneless and skinless), trimmed
¼ tsp. of salt
¼ tsp. black pepper
1 (7 oz.) jar red peppers, rinsed
¼ c. slivered almonds
4 T. extra-virgin olive oil
1 clove of crushed garlic
1 teaspoon paprika
½ tsp. ground cumin
¼ teaspoon crushed red pepper flakes (optional for extra spice)
2 c. cooked quinoa
¼ cup Kalamata olives, diced
¼ cup red onion, minced
1 c. of cucumber, diced
¼ c. crumbled Feta cheese
2 Tbsp. fresh parsley, minced

## **Preparation**

1. Turn on oven broiler at "high" setting, with the rack in the upper third of the oven. Place foil over the top of a baking sheet.

2. Sprinkle the pepper and salt on the chicken breasts and put them on the foil-covered baking sheet. Broil the chicken for 14 to 18 minutes, turning over halfway through the time. They are cooked when the internal temperature (read with a meat thermometer) reads 165 degrees Fahrenheit.

3. Use a sharp knife or forks to slice or shred the cooked chicken breasts on a cutting board.

4. While the chicken cooks, add the following components to a small food processor: half of the oil (2 tablespoons), peppers, garlic, almonds, cumin, paprika, and crushed red pepper flakes (optional). Puree all of these together until they form a relatively smooth sauce.

5. In a medium bowl, add the following components: quinoa, the rest of the olive oil (2 tablespoons), red onion, and olives. Use a large spoon to stir them together.

6. Serve by dividing the quinoa mixture between 4 bowls. Top each bowl with equal amounts of the chicken, cucumber, and red pepper sauce. Over the top, sprinkle parsley and feta cheese.

7. If making this dish ahead of time, store the chicken, sauce, and quinoa mixture in three separate containers and combine just before serving.

8. One serving is 3 oz. of chicken, ¼ c. of the sauce, and ½ c. of the quinoa.

9. Enjoy!

*Low-Carbohydrate Variation:* Use 1 cup of quinoa and 1 ½ pound of chicken.

*Low-Sodium Variation:* Take out the table salt, eliminate the kalamata olives, and substitute part-skim mozzarella cheese for feta cheese.

# Tuscany Tuna Salad in Pita

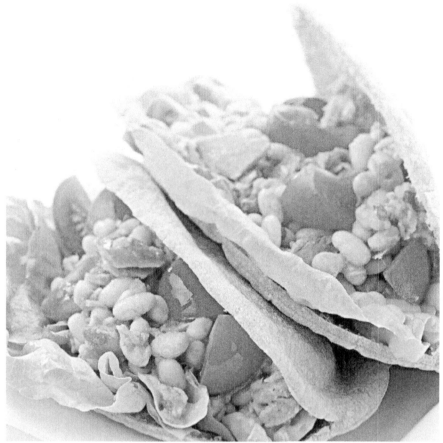

Total Prep and Cooking Time: 10 minutes

## <u>Nutrition (per serving)</u>
Calories: 322
Fat: 9.8 g.
Carbohydrates: 45.1 g.
Protein: 20.7 g.

Serves 4 people

This meal represents a simplified version of a northern Italian dish. It's quick and easy to prepare and can be stored in the refrigerator for a few days. This light but filling fare is also versatile – serve it in a bowl, in a wrap, on a sandwich, or in a pita pocket as this recipe instructs. It's perfect for lunch in the office or a warm summer evening on the porch. The suggested tuna for this salad is chunk light, packed in water, because it is lower in mercury than white albacore tuna and lower in fat than tuna packed in oil.

## Components

2 small cans drained chunk light tuna
4 green onions (scallions), sliced
10 cherry tomatoes, washed and quartered
2 Tbsp. extra virgin olive oil
2 Tbsp. lemon juice
¼ tsp. salt
1 (15 oz.) can of drained and rinsed cannellini beans
ground black pepper, to taste
lettuce leaves, any variety of your choosing
4 pieces of medium pita bread (5 ¼ inch diameter), with pockets inside

## Preparation:

1. Add the following ingredients to a medium bowl: tomatoes, tuna, beans, olive oil, green onions, lemon juice, pepper, and salt. Use a spoon to stir it all together gently. Cover and refrigerate the salad until ready to serve.
2. To serve, line the inside of the pita bread pockets with lettuce and scoop one cup of the tuna salad on top of the lettuce. Enjoy!

*Low-Carbohydrate Variation:* Serve the tuna salad in a lettuce wrap instead of a pita pocket.

*Low-Sodium Variation:* Eliminate the table salt and use "very low sodium" canned white albacore tuna in water instead of chunk light tuna. The white albacore tuna, however, has more mercury, so it is not advisable for pregnant women and for children.

**Beet and Shrimp Salad**

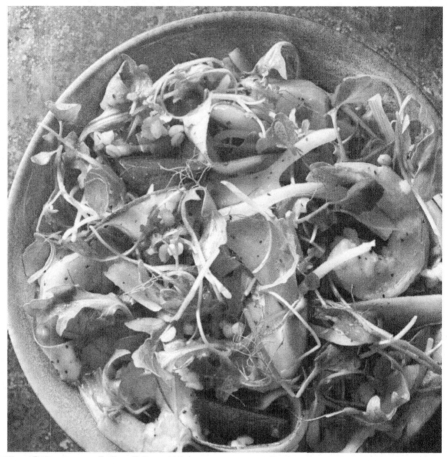

Total Prep and Cooking Time: 15-20 minutes

## <u>Nutrition (per serving)</u>
Calories: 584
Fat: 30 g.
Carbohydrates: 47 g.
Protein: 35 g.

Serves 1 person

At first glance, the amount of fat in this mouth-watering salad may frighten you, but of the 30 grams of fat, only 4 grams is saturated fat! That means that the rest is heart-healthy, appetite-satisfying monounsaturated or polyunsaturated fat. Packed with tasty and nutritious veggies and fiber-full barley, this Beet and Shrimp Salad will brighten up the dreariest day and give you an energy boost that you need to get through your afternoon. This recipe only serves one, but it can easily be doubled, tripled, or even quadrupled when you're serving friends or family.

## Components

2 c. arugula

1 c. watercress

1 c. cooked beet wedges (usually found with other prepared vegetables in your  grocery store's produce  department)

½ c. zucchini ribbons (see step 1 for preparation)

½ c. of thinly sliced fennel

½ c. cooked barley

4 oz. cooked, peeled shrimp (fresh or frozen and thawed)

2 Tbsp. extra-virgin olive oil

1 Tbsp. wine vinegar (red or white, your preference)

½ tsp. mustard (preferably Dijon)

½ teaspoon minced shallot

¼ teaspoon ground pepper

1/8 teaspoon salt

## Preparation

1. To make zucchini ribbons, use a vegetable peeler to shave a whole zucchini lengthwise thinly.
2. On a plate, arrange the watercress, beet wedges, arugula, zucchini ribbons, fennel, shrimp, and barley.
3. Add the following ingredients to a small bowl or bottle: salt, pepper, mustard, minced shallot, olive oil, and wine

vinegar. Combine with a whisk in a bowl or shake in a closed bottle until thoroughly mixed.

4. Drizzle dressing over the salad and enjoy!

*Low-Carbohydrate Variation:* Use half the beets, eliminate the barley, and use 6 ounces of shrimp.

*Low-Sodium Variation:* Eliminate the table salt.

## Italian Veggie Sandwich

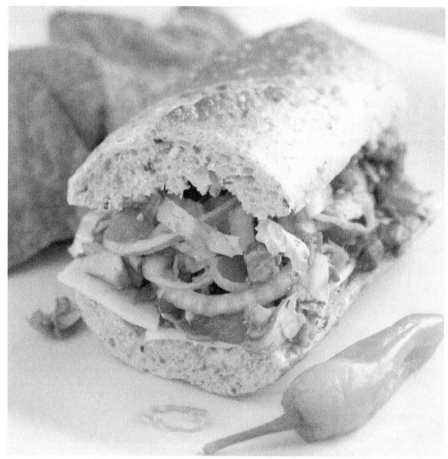

Total Prep and Cooking Time: 20 minutes

## Nutrition (per serving)
Calories: 266
Fat: 8 g.
Carbohydrates: 40 g.

Protein: 14 g.

Serves 4 people

These sub-style sandwiches are a little messy but delightfully zesty and full of fun textures and flavors. They're great for serving at home, on a picnic, or bringing for lunch at the office. One suggestion is to pack the bread and other components separately, then assemble them right before eating. This way, you'll avoid soggy bread! Serve with a salad for even more veggies in your meal.

## Components
¼ c. red onion, thinly sliced, rings separated
1 can of artichoke hearts, rinsed, sliced
1 Roma tomato, diced
1 Tbsp. extra-virgin olive oil
2 Tbsp. balsamic vinegar
1 teaspoon oregano
1 baguette, approximately 20" long, whole grain if possible
2 slices provolone cheese, cut in half
2 c. of romaine lettuce, shredded
¼ c. pepperoncini (optional, for spice)

## Preparation:
1. Place onion rings in a bowl of cold water and set aside while you make the rest of the sandwich.
2. In a medium bowl, place the following components: tomato, artichoke hearts, oregano, oil, vinegar.
3. Cut the baguette into four equivalent portions, then divide them horizontally. Pull out about half the insides from the pieces of bread.
4. Drain the onions from the water and pat dry.
5. For sandwich assembly: place one half-slice of cheese on the bottom half of a baguette portion, then cover with ¼

of the tomato-artichoke mixture. Place ¼ of the lettuce and pepperoncini on top, then place the top half of the baguette upon the sandwich.

6. Serve right away after assembling. Enjoy!

*Low-Carbohydrate Variation:* Serve ingredients in a lettuce wrap or a low-carbohydrate wrap instead of on a baguette.

*Low-Sodium Variation:* Rinse the artichoke hearts thoroughly to eliminate any added salt from the canning juices. Use sliced mozzarella cheese instead of provolone. Do not use the pepperoncini peppers.

# Dinner Selections

## Tomato and Ricotta Whole-Grain Pasta

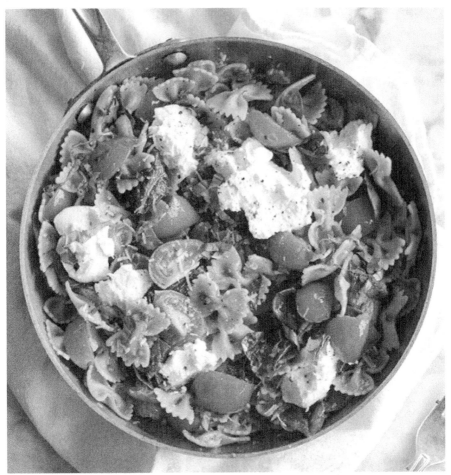

Total Prep and Cooking Time: 25 minutes

## <u>Nutrition (per serving)</u>
Calories: 519
Fat: 29.9 g.
Carbohydrates: 48 g.
Protein: 21.6 g.

Serves 4 people

Although the Mediterranean diet does not contain a whole lot of the carb-heavy pasta most people associate with Italy, there is still a place for whole-grain noodles, eaten in moderation and served with plenty of vegetables! This nutritious dish contains plenty of protein and calcium from ricotta cheese, along with fiber from the whole-wheat pasta. Bright, healthy tomatoes and spinach round out the meal for a flavorful main course that's sure to be a crowd-pleaser. Best of all, it's quick and easy to make.

## Components

8 oz. whole-wheat short pasta (like elbow macaroni, medium shells, or farfalle)
1/3 cup extra-virgin olive oil
3 cloves of garlic, finely minced
8 to 10 cocktail-sized tomatoes, cut into quarters
salt and ground pepper, as much as desired
2 c. fresh leaves of spinach
1/3 c. fresh basil, sliced
½ cup parmesan cheese, grated
1 cup of ricotta cheese

## Preparation:

1. Cook pasta in boiling water for about 1 minute less than package instructions, so pasta is "al dente." Drain, but first set aside ¼ c. of pasta water.
2. Place a large frying pan or sautéing pan on a stove burner. Set to medium and warm up the oil in it. Add the garlic, then set the heat down a little lower. Stir and cook the garlic for five minutes, watching to be sure it doesn't burn, then add the tomatoes. Sprinkle on pepper and salt as desired. Cook an additional 2-3 minutes until tomatoes are warm.
3. In the pan with the tomatoes and garlic, add the cooked pasta and spinach. Use tongs or a large spoon to toss

until the spinach starts wilting gently. Then include the basil, parmesan cheese, and more salt and pepper if desired. Add a little of the pasta water (1-2 tablespoons) or more olive oil if the pasta seems dry at this point.

4. Top the pasta off by dropping scoops of the ricotta cheese on top and serve. Enjoy!

*Low-Carbohydrate Variation:* Use low-carbohydrate pasta. Alternatively, cook and prepare all the ingredients except the pasta. Serve over boneless, skinless chicken breast or fish.

*Low-Sodium Variation:* Use low-sodium pasta.

# Spiced Salmon with Vegetable Quinoa

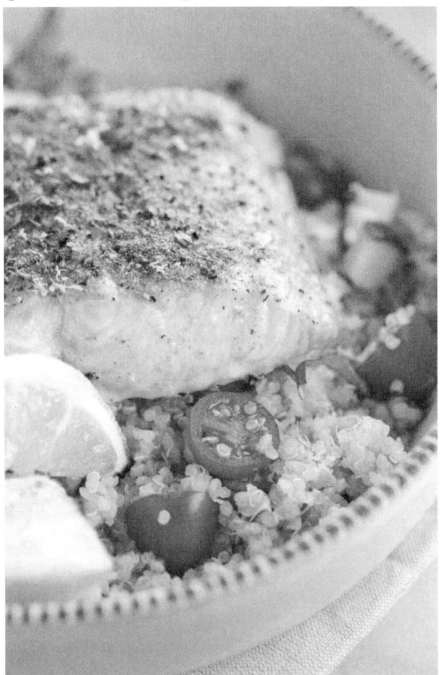

Total Prep and Cooking Time: 30 minutes

## Nutrition (per serving)
Calories: 385
Fat: 12.5 g.
Carbohydrates: 32.5 g.
Protein: 35.5 g.

Serves 4 people

This dish looks so fancy you'd expect it could be served at a restaurant, but the truth is that you can whip it up in just a half hour. The salmon is perfectly seasoned for a combination of heat and pure flavor, and the quinoa is livened up with bright vegetables. The best part is that this dish packs a punch of a whopping 35 grams of protein! What a way to finish off your day.

## Components
1 c. uncooked quinoa
1 tsp. of salt, divided in half
¾ c. cucumbers, seeds removed, diced
1 c. of cherry tomatoes, halved
¼ c. red onion, minced
4 fresh basil leaves, cut in thin slices
zest from one lemon
¼ teaspoon black pepper
1 teaspoon cumin
½ teaspoon paprika
4 (5-oz.) salmon fillets
8 lemon wedges
¼ c. fresh parsley, chopped

## Preparation:
1. To a medium-sized saucepan, add the quinoa, 2 cups of water, and ½ tsp. of the salt. Heat these until the water is boiling, then lower the temperature until it is simmering.

Cover the pan and let it cook 20 minutes or as long as the quinoa package instructs.

2. Turn off the burner under the quinoa and allow it to sit, covered, for at least another 5 minutes before serving.

3. Right before serving, add the onion, tomatoes, cucumbers, basil leaves, and lemon zest to the quinoa and use a spoon to stir everything together gently.

4. In the meantime (while the quinoa cooks), prepare the salmon. Turn on the oven broiler to high and make sure a rack is in the lower part of the oven.

5. To a small bowl, add the following components: black pepper, ½ tsp. of the salt, cumin, and paprika. Stir them together.

6. Place foil over the top of a glass or aluminum baking sheet, then spray it with nonstick cooking spray.

7. Place salmon fillets on the foil. Rub the spice mixture over the surface of each fillet (about ½ tsp. of the spice mixture per fillet).

8. Add the lemon wedges to the pan edges near the salmon.

9. Cook the salmon under the broiler for 8-10 minutes. Your goal is for the salmon to flake apart easily with a fork.

10. Sprinkle the salmon with the parsley, then serve it with the lemon wedges and vegetable parsley. Enjoy!

*Low-Carbohydrate Variation:* Substitute wilted spinach leaves for half the quinoa. Increase the size of the salmon fillets, if desired.

*Low-Sodium Variation:* Eliminate the table salt.

# Easy Lamb Kofta with Chickpeas and Naan

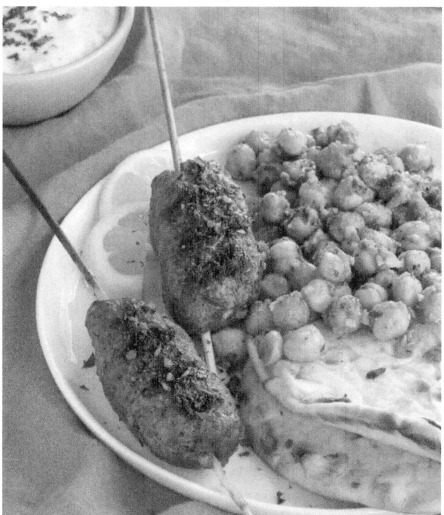

Total Prep and Cooking Time: 60 minutes

## <u>Nutrition (per serving)</u>
Calories: 601
Fat: 38 g.
Carbohydrates: 38 g.
Protein: 30 g.

Serves 4 people

Although at first glance this meal seems a bit heavy on the calories, the numbers you see above include the side dishes as well. This meal is perfectly balanced between fat, protein, and carbohydrates, which makes it entirely satisfying and nutritious. While healthy followers of the Mediterranean diet don't eat red meat very often, there is indeed room for the occasional Greek-style lamb *kofta* (meatball) kebobs! Served with a fresh yogurt sauce, a simple side of sautéed chickpeas with harissa paste (easily found in the ethnic section of most grocery stores), and a small portion of naan (Indian flatbread), this meal is deceptively simple to make. Your guests or family will think you slaved in the kitchen for hours, but you'll know it was a matter of an hour or less.

## Components
*For the kofta*
3 T. red onion, finely minced
3 T. mixed fresh Italian herbs (like parsley, mint, and cilantro), finely minced
3 minced cloves of garlic
1 ¼ teaspoon salt
1 teaspoon cumin
¾ teaspoon paprika
½ teaspoon black pepper
1 lb. ground lamb (ask for the lean ground lamb to minimize saturated fat; can substitute lean ground beef)
nonstick cooking spray
skewers for cooking the meat

*For the sauce*
½ c. plain nonfat yogurt
1 tsp. mixed fresh Italian herbs, finely minced
2 tsp. fresh lemon juice
pinch of salt

*For the chickpeas*

4 Tbsp. extra-virgin olive oil, divided in half

1 T. red onion, minced

1 garlic clove, minced

1 can chickpeas, rinsed and drained

1 tsp. harissa paste (North African hot sauce, found in Mediterranean section of grocery stores)

¾ tsp. of ground cumin

½ tsp. of paprika

salt, to taste

¼ c. low-sodium chicken stock

1 teaspoon lemon juice

1 T. mixed fresh Italian herbs, finely minced

*For serving*

1 store-bought flatbread or naan, preferably whole-wheat, divided into 4 pieces

## **Preparation:**

*Note: You'll notice that the chickpeas, sauce, and kofta all have the same Italian herbs in them. You can save time by chopping all the herbs together ahead of time, instead of individually for each dish.

1. *Prepare the kofta meat:* In a stand mixer's bowl, add all the kofta components except the meat itself. Mix on slow speed with a beater blade until these parts are combined. Then incorporate the meat by beating until thoroughly combined with the other parts. Use plastic wrap to cover this bowl and refrigerate it until ready to cook the meat. Meanwhile, prepare the rest of the dishes.

2. When ready to cook the meat, grab a handful and form it into an oblong, sausage-like shape (see picture), then stick a skewer through it. You can also make any other shape you like with the meat – patties, meatballs, etc.- and you do not have to use skewers.

3. Set a large pan or griddle on med-high heat and spray it generously with nonstick cooking spray. When the surface is very hot, cook the meat skewers for 3 to 4 minutes per side, until deep golden on both sides and cooked thoroughly.

4. *Make the yogurt sauce:* Within a bowl, place yogurt, herbs, lemon juice, and salt. Use a whisk or spoon to stir thoroughly and set aside.

5. *Cook the chickpeas:* Set a large sautéing pan on the stove over a burner set to medium. Heat up 2 Tbsp. of the oil, then cook the onions in the heated oil for one to two minutes, until they become just softened. Then incorporate the garlic and sauté for another thirty seconds.

6. Next, add the harissa, chickpeas, paprika, cumin, salt, and chicken stock. Increase the heat under the pan to high and cook while stirring until almost all the stock has evaporated.

7. Remove pan from heat and add the lemon juice and herbs, then stir. Add the rest of the oil right before you serve it.

8. *To serve:* Divide meatballs and chickpeas among 4 plates. Add a ¼ piece of naan or whole-wheat flatbread to each plate. Serve with yogurt sauce for dipping or drizzling over meatballs. Enjoy!

Low-Carbohydrate Variation: Serve a salad or sautéed vegetables instead of chickpeas. Eliminate the flatbread.

Low-Sodium Variation: Eliminate the table salt. Use unsalted chicken broth instead of low-sodium chicken broth.

# Slow-Cooker Mediterranean Chicken with Quinoa

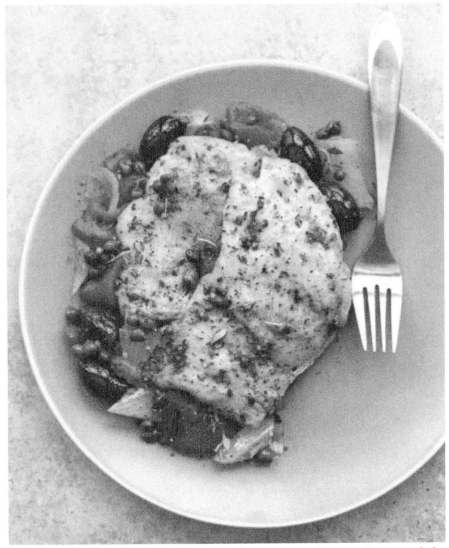

Total Prep and Cooking Time: 4 hours, 5 minutes (most of the time is inactive, while chicken cooks in the slow cooker)

## Nutrition (per serving; with quinoa)
Calories: 356
Fat: 11 grams
Carbohydrates: 35 grams
Protein: 30.2 grams

## Nutrition (per serving; without quinoa)
Calories: 200
Fat: 8.6 g.
Carbohydrates: 7.6 g.
Protein: 24.2 g.

Serves 4 people

You've got to love the slow cooker concept – start a meal in the morning or the middle of the day, go about your business, and voila! You have dinner when you come home later. The convenience of this kitchen gadget cannot be overstated, not to mention the joy of coming home to the wonderful smells of dinner already cooking. This simple but delicious dish combines classic Mediterranean flavors with the lean protein of boneless, skinless chicken breasts. Serve it with some quinoa, and you've got a complete meal! This is an easy dish that will quickly become a family favorite.

## Components:
nonstick cooking spray
4 medium chicken breasts (boneless and skinless; about 4 oz. each)
salt and pepper, as much as desired
3 tsp. Italian seasoning
2 Tbsp. lemon juice
1 Tbsp. garlic, minced
1 medium onion, roughly chopped
1 c. kalamata olives
1 c. jarred red peppers, drained, diced
2 T. capers
fresh basil or thyme for garnish (optional)
1 cup uncooked quinoa

## Preparation:

1. Sprinkle pepper and salt over the chicken breasts. Warm a skillet on stove burner over med-low heat and cook chicken for one or two minutes on each side, or just until becoming brown.

2. Spray inside the slow cooker with nonstick spray and put in the browned chicken breasts. Add olives, capers, red peppers, and onion around the sides of the breasts, not over the top.

3. Within a bowl, place the following components: lemon juice, Italian seasoning, and garlic. Use a whisk to combine them. Pour this mixture over the components of the slow cooker.

4. Cover the slow cooker; cook on low heat for 4 hours. You can also cook it on high for 2 hours.

5. When it is almost time for dinner, cook the quinoa according to package directions.

6. To serve, divide the quinoa among 4 plates, then top with one chicken breast on each plate. Divide the rest of the crockpot ingredients between the 4 plates and serve. Enjoy!

*Low-Carbohydrate Variation:* Serve on a bed of greens instead of quinoa. Use more chicken if desired.

*Low-Sodium Variation:* Eliminate the table salt and kalamata olives.

# Speedy Shrimp Puttanesca

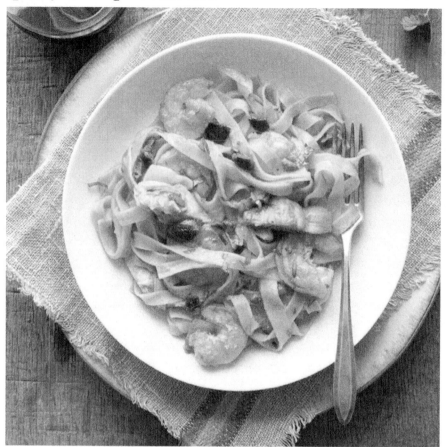

Total Prep and Cooking Time: 15 minutes

## Nutrition (per serving)
Calories: 390
Fat: 8 g.
Carbohydrates: 43 g.
Protein: 37 g.

Serves 4 people

Fresh pasta (found in the refrigerated section of your grocery store) cooks much faster than dried pasta so the dish can be on your table swiftly! Puttanesca is usually made with anchovies, capers, olives, tomatoes, and garlic; however, here it gets a protein boost from the shrimp and a fiber boost from artichokes. You'll love the flavor combination and the ease with which you can prepare this meal for yourself and your family.

## Components

8 oz. fresh refrigerated linguini noodles, whole-wheat if possible
1 T. extra-virgin olive oil
1 pound peeled, deveined large shrimp (fresh or frozen and thawed)
1 medium can of tomato sauce, without added salt
1 ¼ c. artichoke hearts, quartered (purchase frozen or canned; drain if canned)
¼ c. Kalamata olives, pitted and chopped
1 T. capers, rinsed
¼ tsp. of salt

## Preparation:

1. Place a large pot of water on a stove burner set on high and heat until the water is boiling. Cook the linguini as the package instructs, and then drain.
2. Pour the oil in a large sautéing pan and heat it on high. Place shrimp in hot oil in a single layer. Cook them without moving them for 2 to 3 minutes until the bottoms are browned. Then stir the tomato sauce in and add the capers, salt, olives, and artichoke hearts. Keep stirring and cooking this mixture for 2 to 3 more minutes, until shrimp are thoroughly cooked, and the artichoke hearts are hot.
3. To the sauce, add the drained cooked noodles and mix together.
4. To serve, divide the noodles and sauce between 4 plates or bowls. Enjoy!

*Low-Carbohydrate Variation:* Use cooked spaghetti squash or cooked zucchini ribbons instead of linguini.

*Low-Sodium Variation:* Eliminate the table salt and kalamata olives.

## Appetizer/Snack Selections

### Flatbread Pizza with Spinach and White Bean Pesto

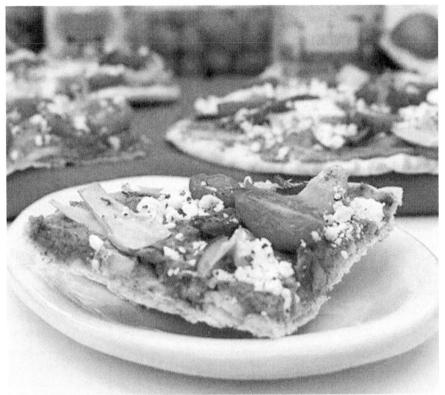

Total Prep and Cooking Time: 20 minutes

### Nutrition (per ½ flatbread for an appetizer; double for whole flatbread as a meal)
Calories: 225
Fat: 9.5 g.
Carbohydrates: 28.5 g.
Protein: 8.5 g.

Serves 6 people for an appetizer or 3 people for a meal

If you have an intense desire for a pizza, rejoice! There's a nutritious, relatively guilt-free option that fits well in your Mediterranean eating plan. These delicious little flatbread pizzas should satisfy your craving without adding to your waistline. They're great as a main dish for a Friday night meal or served as an appetizer at a party. This dish piles on the produce, and the white bean and spinach pesto give this dish a unique flavor that will have your guests clamoring for more.

## Components:

3 pieces of naan or pita bread (about 78 g. each, preferably whole-wheat)

2/3 c. canned cannellini or great northern beans, rinsed and drained

2 cups of spinach

1 Tbsp. Extra-Virgin olive oil

¼ cup raw natural almonds

¼ c. fresh basil, torn into pieces

2 T. water

¼ teaspoon salt, and additional for sprinkling

1/8 teaspoon black pepper

½ c. of cherry or grape tomatoes halved

½ c. marinated artichoke hearts, roughly chopped

½ of a medium avocado, sliced thinly

¼ small red onion, sliced thinly

2 oz. feta cheese with Mediterranean herbs

## Preparation:

1. Turn on oven and set to 350 degrees Fahrenheit. On a baking sheet, place the 3 pieces of pita bread or naan.
2. In a food processor, add the following components: salt, pepper, water, basil, white beans, spinach, almonds, and basil. Pulse to puree until almost entirely smooth. Using a spoon, spread this pesto evenly on the pieces of bread.
3. Arrange the following on top of the pesto: onion slices, avocado slices, chopped artichoke hearts, and halved

tomatoes. Sprinkle the cheese and a little salt over the top of each.

4. Place pan in the oven and leave it to bake for approximately 10 minutes, or until bread is crispy. Let it cool off slightly, then slice each flatbread into 4 pieces with a pizza cutter. Serve and enjoy!

_Low-Carbohydrate Variation:_ Serve toppings on a low-carb crust or make a crust from pureed cauliflower.

_Low-Sodium Variation:_ Eliminate the table salt. Substitute mozzarella for feta cheese. Use canned or frozen artichoke hearts instead of marinated.

# Turkey Meatballs with Yogurt Herb Dip

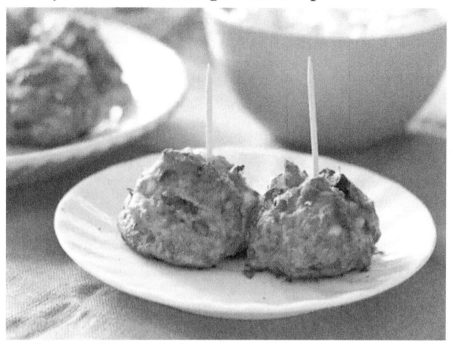

Total Prep and Cooking Time: 50 minutes

## Nutrition (per 2 meatballs)
Calories: 157
Fat: 6.6 g.
Carbohydrates: 11.9 g.
Protein: 12.7 g.

The recipe makes 20 (2" diameter) meatballs.

These delightful little meatballs have a surprising twist – they have lentils, feta, and a few other unusual ingredients inside, the result of which is a perfect savory appetizer. In case you're wondering, they'd also be perfect in a batch of marinara sauce on pasta or mixed up with greens for a protein-packed salad. Although they're hardly traditional, they contain several critical elements of the Mediterranean diet.

## Components

*For the meatballs*

1 c. lentils, already cooked (black or green)

½ lb. ground turkey

2 lg. eggs, beaten

2/3 cup breadcrumbs

½ c. part-skim ricotta

¼ c. feta cheese crumbles

2 Tbsp. red onion, minced

2 Tbsp. black olives, chopped

1 Tbsp. capers

2 Tbsp. Italian parsley, minced

½ teaspoon oregano

¼ teaspoon dried dill

½ teaspoon of salt


*For the yogurt dip*

1 c. Greek yogurt (plain, nonfat)

1 clove of garlic, minced

½ teaspoon chives, fresh or dried

1 tsp. chopped dill, fresh or dried

1 teaspoon lemon juice

salt and pepper, as much as desired


## Preparation:

1. Use a food processor to pulse cooked lentils until they have the consistency of mush, then move them from the food processor and place within a bowl. Then add the rest of the meatball components to the mushed-up lentils. Use your hands, a spatula, or a spoon to mix it all together thoroughly. Allow this mixture to rest for 15 minutes.

2. Heat up the oven and set it to 375 degrees Fahrenheit. Prepare a baking sheet with parchment paper or non-stick spray. Form 20 meatballs by hand from the

meatball mixture and place them on the prepared baking sheet. They can be fairly close together because they don't spread out much.

3.  Place the sheet of meatballs on the middle rack of the heated oven and bake them 20-22 minutes. They should be golden brown before you take them out of the oven. Allow them to cool off outside the oven.

4.  While the meatballs bake, make the yogurt dip. Add all the components of the sauce to a small bowl and whisk them together until thoroughly combined. Cover the bowl and chill until ready to serve.

5.  Keep meatballs and yogurt in the refrigerator until ready to serve. The meatballs will keep for 3 to 4 days, and the dip will keep for 7 to 10 days.

6.  Enjoy!

_Low-Carbohydrate Variation:_ This is a low-carb recipe. You can use more lentils and fewer breadcrumbs if you like, but this may change the texture too much.

_Low-Sodium Variation:_ Eliminate the table salt. Use mozzarella instead of feta cheese.

# Garlicy Spanish Shrimp

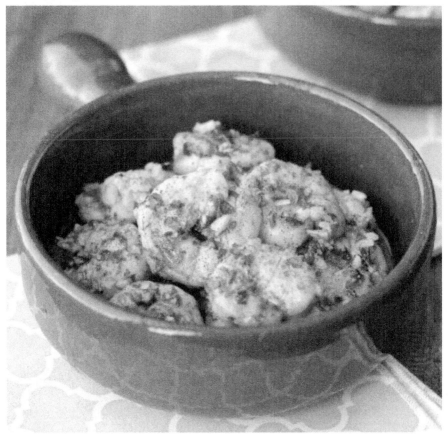

Total Prep and Cooking Time: 15 minutes

## Nutrition (per ¼ recipe)
Calories: 250
Fat: 17.9 g.
Carbohydrates: 3.4 g.
Protein: 15.8 g.

Recipe serves 4 or more people.

Hardly anything beats shrimp when it comes to versatility and
flavor delivered in a small package. This dish mimics the idea of
Spanish *tapas* – small dishes designed to be shared between a

few people. If you add toothpicks to the shrimp, you have a perfect snack or before-dinner appetizer. A bonus is all the nutrition packed into this dish. Shrimp deliver a large dose of selenium, which is an important nutrient for your immune system and heart. The olive oil adds some heart-healthy monounsaturated fat as well.

## Components:
1/3 cup extra-virgin olive oil
4 cloves of garlic, minced
¼ teaspoon chili flakes
1 lb. large shrimp, deveined and peeled
1 teaspoon paprika
¼ teaspoon salt
1/8 teaspoon black pepper
2 Tbsp. dry sherry
1 ½ Tbsp. lemon juice
2 Tbsp. fresh parsley, chopped

## Preparation:
1. To a large sautéing pan, add the oil, garlic and chili flakes. Set the heat under the pan to medium-high. Heating the oil with the garlic and chili will infuse the oil with these flavors. Be sure not to let the garlic brown.
2. After the oil becomes hot, place the shrimp in the pan and sprinkle the paprika, salt, and pepper over them. Stir the pan often while the shrimp cook for two minutes, until starting to turn pink.
3. Add the sherry and lemon juice to the pan. Keep stirring and cooking for another 2-3 minutes or until the shrimp are cooked through, and the liquid has reduced.
4. Sprinkle the parsley on top of the shrimp and serve. Enjoy!
5.

*Low-Carbohydrate Variation:* This is a low-carbohydrate recipe.

*Low-Sodium Variation:* Eliminate the table salt.

## Italian-Style Roasted Veggies and Mushrooms

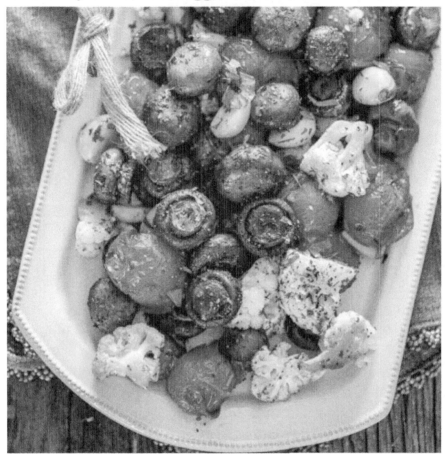

Total Prep and Cooking Time: 30 minutes

### Nutrition (in each serving)
Calories: 87
Fat: 4 grams
Carbohydrates: 9 grams
Protein: 3 grams

Serves 6 people.

This simple dish makes a great appetizer or side dish. It's full of colorful, nutritious vegetables and sure to be a hit. Because it is so quick and easy to prepare, you'll love bringing it along to your next potluck party. Your waistline will appreciate the low-calorie count, too!

## Components:
1 lb. cremini mushrooms, cleaned
2 c. cauliflower, cut into small florets
2 c. cocktail tomatoes
12 cloves garlic, peeled
2 Tbsp. extra-virgin olive oil
1 Tbsp. Italian seasoning
salt and pepper, as much as desired
1 T. fresh parsley, chopped

## Preparation:
1. Turn on oven and set it to 400 degrees Fahrenheit.
2. Place all the mushrooms and vegetables within a bowl. Then include the olive oil, Italian seasoning, salt, and pepper. Use a spoon to toss until all these components are combined gently.
3. Spread contents of the bowl out on a sheet for baking and place it in the hot oven. Allow vegetables and mushrooms to roast 20 or 30 minutes. Make sure that the mushrooms are golden-brown (but not burnt) and the cauliflower can be easily pierced by a fork.
4. Sprinkle chopped fresh parsley over the dish just before serving. Enjoy!

*Low-Carbohydrate Variation:* The only carbohydrates in this dish come from vegetables, which cannot be eliminated without changing the recipe entirely.

*Low-Sodium Variation:* Eliminate the table salt.

# Antipasto Skewers

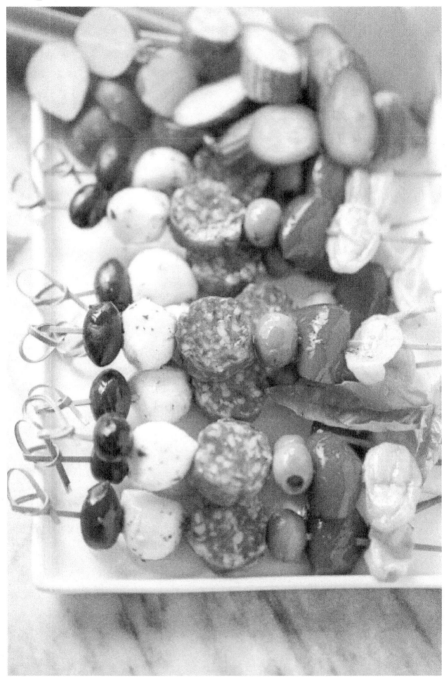

Total Prep and Cooking Time: 6 minutes

## Nutrition (per skewer)

Calories: 55
Fat: 4 g.
Carbohydrates: 1 g.
Protein: 2 g.

The recipe makes 12 skewers.

These delicious and adorable little skewers take mere minutes to assemble, and they are sure to be a hit at your next party! They contain all the essential flavors of a Mediterranean diet, plus their small size makes portion control a cinch. The strong taste and unique texture of each bite are sure to satisfy you and your guests.

## Components:

12 of each of the following

- kalamata olives, pitted
- mozzarella cheese balls
- small thick slices of salami
- pimento-stuffed green olives
- halves of jarred cherry peppers (6 peppers, cut in half)
- small pepperoncini peppers

## Preparation:

1. Use 12 7-inch skewers. Stick one of each component on each skewer in any order of your choosing.
2. Store skewers in the refrigerator until ready to serve. These can be stored for up to a day.
3. Serve and enjoy!

*Low-Carbohydrate Variation:* This is a low-carb recipe.

*Low-Sodium Variation:* Unfortunately, most of the components of this recipe have a high level of sodium, so it is best to avoid this appetizer.

# Conclusion

Thank for making it through to the end of *"Mediterranean Diet for Beginners."* Let's hope it was informative and able to provide you with all of the tools you need to achieve your healthy lifestyle goals.

By reading this book, you have made an essential first step in the exciting journey towards better health and a celebration of living with a fresh new approach to food. Now, you have the secret to why so many people around the Mediterranean Sea are living long, healthy, and happy lives surrounded by family members and friends. So, what are you going to do now that you know the secret?

The next step is to get cooking! Start shopping and cooking as soon as possible. You are likely eager to try some of the delicious recipes you read in this guide. If you are looking for more support, there are thousands of people online and throughout your community who have also embraced the Mediterranean lifestyle, and they will be eager to support you as you explore this new way of eating and approaching life. You'll also want to lace up your walking shoes and start getting active today. The sooner you start, the closer you'll be to achieving your goals of establishing and maintaining a healthy new lifestyle. You are at an exciting new place in life, so enjoy every moment of it!

Finally, if you found this book useful in any way, a review on Amazon is always appreciated!

# Other books by Serena Baker

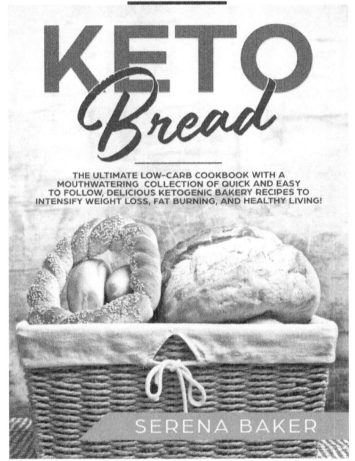

## Keto Bread

*Low Carb Keto Bread Recipes!*

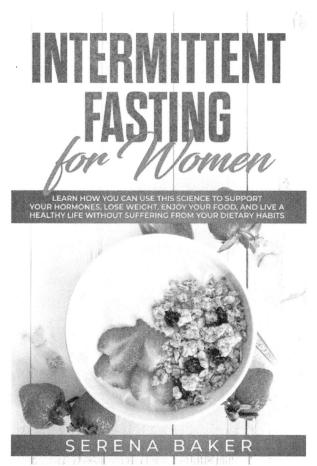

# Intermittent Fasting For Women

*Intermittent Fasting designed specifically for Women*

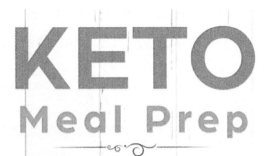

# KETO
## Meal Prep

**QUICK, HEALTHY AND DELICIOUS
READY-TO-GO KETOGENIC DIET MEALS
TO PREP THAT ACTUALLY TASTE GOOD**

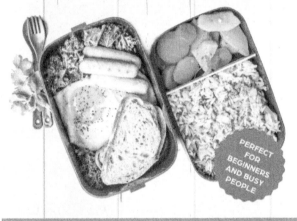

PERFECT FOR BEGINNERS AND BUSY PEOPLE

**SERENA BAKER**

# *Keto Meal Prep*

*Healthy and delicious ketogenic diet meals to prep,
grab, and go!*

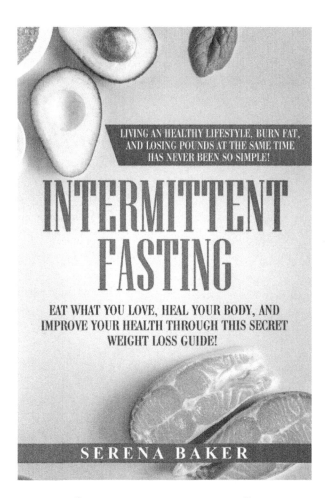

LIVING AN HEALTHY LIFESTYLE, BURN FAT, AND LOSING POUNDS AT THE SAME TIME HAS NEVER BEEN SO SIMPLE!

# INTERMITTENT FASTING

EAT WHAT YOU LOVE, HEAL YOUR BODY, AND IMPROVE YOUR HEALTH THROUGH THIS SECRET WEIGHT LOSS GUIDE!

SERENA BAKER

# *Intermittent Fasting: The Guide*

*The best guide on Intermittent Fasting*

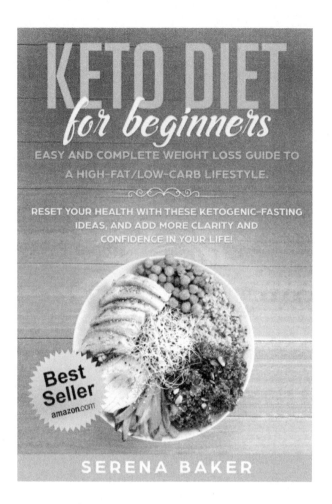

# Keto Diet For Beginners: The Guide

*The best guide on the Keto Diet*

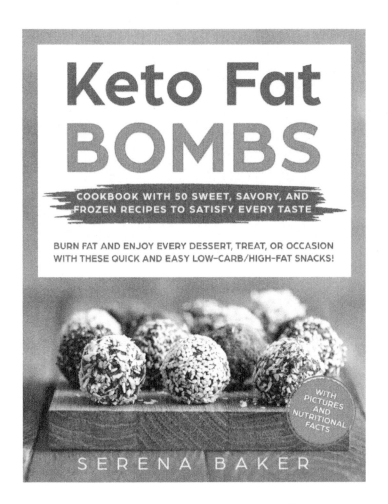

# Keto Fat Bombs

*A collection of 50 mouthwatering keto recipes*

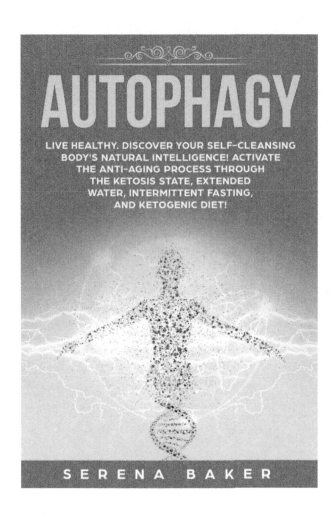

# *Autophagy*

*Discover your self-cleansing body's natural intelligence!*

Printed in Great Britain
by Amazon

81903049R00081